# LIFE and DEATH

# LIFE and DEATH

The History of Overcoming Disease and
What It Tells Us About Our Present Increasing
Life Expectancy as a Result
of Present Day Actions

## *John Durbin Husher*

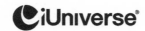

# LIFE AND DEATH
## The History of Overcoming Disease and What It Tells Us About Our Present Increasing Life Expectancy as a Result of Present Day Actions

iUniverse books may be ordered through booksellers or by contacting:

iUniverse
1663 Liberty Drive
Bloomington, IN 47403
www.iuniverse.com
1-800-Authors (1-800-288-4677)

Because of the dynamic nature of the Internet, any web addresses or links contained in this book may have changed since publication and may no longer be valid. The views expressed in this work are solely those of the author and do not necessarily reflect the views of the publisher, and the publisher hereby disclaims any responsibility for them.

Any people depicted in stock imagery provided by Thinkstock are models, and such images are being used for illustrative purposes only. Certain stock imagery © Thinkstock.

ISBN: 978-1-4917-7780-0 (sc)
ISBN: 978-1-4917-8678-9 (hc)
ISBN: 978-1-4917-7779-4 (e)

Library of Congress Control Number: 2015915231

Print information available on the last page.

iUniverse rev. date: 01/04/2016

# Introduction

The book *Life and Death* covers both of these subjects, but it is mainly about life and living and the individual doctors and bio scientists who struggled to increase human life. This set the stage for actions that are proceeding as you read this book. There is no stopping the medical community and the technical community that support today's medical advances. The reader will find it exciting, after reviewing the past, how much is being done today on a daily basis. The reader will find it exciting to read the details on the five major catastrophes that caused the loss of hundreds of millions of human lives, and further on in the book I cover why I don't expect any of these catastrophic events to be repeated.

The major contributions to extending life are covered beginning in the eighteenth century with several key inventions and the constant energy applied to learning about life by key individuals. You will enjoy reading about each of these individuals and how they proceeded to make their marks on human history. Several technological advances during this time period aided the bio scientists in their quest to overcome death-causing phenomena. Although this is history, it sets the stage for today's continuing battle against disease, further learning about the human body, and major technical advances that carry us forward in the battle. These more recent advances will be helpful to those who want to understand what is available today.

As a result of the discovery of the microscope, the war on disease went from a defensive one to one where humanity was on the offensive. Investigators could now see the "beasties" that were causing the problems, and his studies went from those that were sick, to one where the bio scientists were after the cause to prevent future sickness. The reader will be excited to learn of the medical advances presently being pursued by our scientists, bio scientists, doctors, and technical support efforts by major scientific firms. Present-day efforts are producing many new discoveries and medical advances that affect today's people, including advances for children and new findings and cures for young adults and older adults over eighty years old.

By the turn of the twentieth century, major impacts had been made to the extension of life but there was still no understanding of how to deal with the major diseases, such as streptococcus and staphylococcus. Man could now see them, but there was no immediate answer as to how to prevent their destruction on life. After World War I there was a major impact on dealing with these and other diseases. Now one reads about the development of the first vaccines to attack and prevent many of the culprits. You will be excited by the war that developed on cures for diseases discovered in the twentieth century and continues on in the first fifteen years of this century.

Still, it was not known what made man function as he does. The search had been on since the beginning of time as to how a person is conceived and why each one of us is different from any other one. The search was on for the genetic code and the secret of life. The bio scientists had their initial thoughts, and when those didn't work out they searched in different directions for the answers to life. It's exciting to see how an American and three English scientists found the answers during the middle of the twentieth century. Their findings led them to the genetic code and understanding the code. They found DNA and RNA and how one worked with the other. This sets the stage for today's major impacts on life and many of today's cures and the continuous look for what the near future holds for us.

Follow through the scientific research that took the bio scientists' steps from the code to the human genome and beyond. Now one could begin to review the genome of many species, how the various parts of the genome interact with each other, and possible cures with this knowledge. These are discussed on the up-to-date effects that are expanding and taking on today's medical issues. The readers will be interested in possible impacts on their lives and the lives of their children and their friends.

And then there are new diseases that maim or kill many. Along came HIV and AIDS and the search for the cause and the search for the cure—if not a cure, maybe a delay. You will read how bio scientists had learned much from how DNA and RNA work, and how this gave them significant information on how HIV, AIDS, and hepatitis C work, along with today's work on solutions. Anyone with these diseases will be quite interested in finding what is being done on a daily basis to overcome each of these and other massive diseases.

The twentieth century, mainly after World War I, resulted in bio scientists beginning to make major impacts on diseases and the prevention of them through vaccines. Many vaccines were discovered and invoked across the world. Details of the vaccines bring out many interesting facts and reactions. Many new medications were developed, and this book covers many that are presently used and those that provide even more help. Details are covered on many new findings that will be miracle cures for today's population—and they continue on a daily basis. Perhaps there is an answer for one of the readers to find something about problems they have and the medications presently available as well as the vaccines to help each of you. One will see that even though there may not be an answer today for their problems that an answer may only be a short time away.

Today there are outbreaks of many of the diseases that were previously solved by using vaccines; now those diseases are erupting in various countries, including the United States. Read why this is happening and what it takes to get back to stable results on those diseases. Anyone interested in understanding today's actions to overcome these diseases will find exciting details about many of them.

Read about how we should be able to prevent any of the world's previous big killers of humans. Remember the five major catastrophes that are discussed earlier in this book; these are reviewed for today's answers. But what about Ebola, which is now killing many people each week in three countries in northwestern Africa? The reader will be amazed at the present-day actions taken to prevent the spread of these type of medical problems to today's population and the cures developed during this year for the problems.

Late in the twentieth century bio scientists found the stem cell and its reactions within a human being. In the first decade of this century they found adult stem cells and how both the embryonic stem cells and adult stem cells could be the next answer to solving life-threatening disease or solving lifelong torturous ailments—perhaps not curing them but making them bearable. Here were new answers to what might be needed to solve today's major medical issues—a more detailed understanding of human life. Readers interested in the technical details of today's adventures on DNA, the human genome, and stem cells will find many significant points to review.

You will read about the fantastic results on the solutions that provided a continuous increase of the average life span and implications of the future great expansion of the average life span for people all over the world … from when there were three hundred million inhabitants on earth to the present number of over seven billion and how long they are expected to live. The increased life span is covered right up to today's results, and one will find it exciting to realize how fortunate we are.

Although the early stages of this book demonstrate how man historically began to take over the control of life; readers will be highly interested in what today's actions hold for each of them.

# Table of Contents

# *Overview*

Life on earth can be evolutionary and lasting for many years before normal death, or it can be suddenly culminated by an unnatural death. In this book I chose to call unnatural death as non-evolutionary, which is one that is caused by an outside event such as murder, a war, or a massive disease, and happens in a very short and unexpected time. This book covers the evolutionary advances of medicine and brings one up-to-date on today's immediate actions.

Over the years the average life span has been increasing, and one of the purposes of this book is to show the tenacity and innovation it took to affect this increase. Consider that the average life span of a person in the United States was just over twenty seven two hundred years ago. The average life span was low due to a host of limiting factors, mostly medical, many of which have been dramatically reduced over the last two hundred years. There have also been many technical issues that had to be overcome, and this book covers many of those innovations right up to the present time. As a result of these reductions the average life span has dramatically increased over the past two hundred years. A prime example shows that not as long ago as the early 1700s in the United States a person was fortunate to live beyond the age of twenty-nine. During the nineteenth and twentieth centuries we saw a very dramatic rise in this average life span. The focus on things such as the food we ate, clean city water for cities, reduction in infant mortality, frequent cleaning of the hands, and understanding what caused early death were quite effective in leading to medical intervention and the resulting successful medical evolution. Some of the medical evolution was the result of serendipity, as will be discussed; but the main improvements were due to skillful, tenacious, hardworking, and patient stubbornness displayed by those who practiced some form of medical work. Medical intervention resulted in improvements in health followed by subsequent improvements carrying the initial discoveries to the next complex step in the evolution. This medical revolution continues right up to the present time and includes advances in today's technical equipment and communication equipment that speed up medical actions.

**Technical innovations were also instrumental in allowing new methods to be utilized in much of the new medical industry. These will be discussed as to how they improve medical intervention. Time and significant subsequent innovative steps resulted in the average life span in the United States increasing to above the mid-seventies early in the twenty-first century. Data indicate it will continue to rise. Worldwide data show that several countries have increased their country's average life span to even higher levels than the United States.** [1]

One of purposes of this writing is to cover the individuals who contributed significantly to this increase in one's life span as well as their unbelievable tenacity and innovation that occurred to carry significant findings to the next step. You will find discussions about each of these individuals and their intense devotion to finding causes and cures, as well as the impact that resulted in each of these cases.

One-third into the book I bring the reader to the present time span, and I have detailed many of the medical advances over the last one hundred years—right up to July 2015. These include the enormous amounts of vaccines that have revolutionized the medical world and how they have spread to many of the large and poorer economies in the world. Anyone presently suffering from a medical problem or a disease should read these sections for inputs that may help you. Technical advances in the instrumentation of equipment to handle medical problems in a more defined manner are discussed. These include the technical advances in present-day communication equipment that allow almost instant realization across all the countries of the world.

Meanwhile, there also were many non-evolutionary deaths in large numbers of people over the years, and especially during the fourteenth and twentieth centuries. These deaths were mainly those imposed by dramatic charges by man on man that resulted in wars invoking massive deaths or through dramatic life-taking disease or starvation phenomena that caused a huge number of people to lose their lives. There were many of these significant death-causing incidents over the course of time, but I will identify the five worse ones and detail their marked effects on life in this world we live in. A later section of this book covers the present actions installed to prevent reoccurrence of these types of events.

One of the purposes of this writing is to review the evolutionary steps that have been discovered over the years to increase man's life span and increase the overall population of the world, as well as to review how large numbers were lost to non-evolutionary means. A focus on each of these areas is worth reviewing to portray the tremendous understanding and invention that was involved to positively affect the evolutionary growth, while reviewing how the sudden impacts of the non-evolutionary areas affected the growth in the negative direction and came close to preventing sanity, and life itself, from prevailing. The reader will see the average life span of man increasing on a rather continuous basis only to fall back due to life-taking phenomena, and then to pick up as the battle is renewed to overcome human failure. It is truly a battle, and one of the purposes of this book is to cover the daily occurrences happening in this twenty-first century.

To provide one overall picture of the magnitude we will be reviewing, consider that the population of the world was just over six hundred million people in 1700. The population in early 2015 is estimated to be over seven billion (7,300,000,000), for a huge growth over 214 years despite numerous deaths due to wars and disease, which will be discussed.

# Non evolutionary Death—
# War and Disease

I have chosen to review non evolutionary death first since it will provide the reader a good background for understanding the basic phenomena that limited growth recently in the world's history. Chronologically this makes sense, since most of this damage was done just prior to the major implementation of the evolutionary increases in life expectancy. It also serves to demonstrate to the reader how tenuous life on earth is and how close we have come to its elimination by recent natural events and events put into motion by man. Many of the people I talked to, or communicated through e-mails with, didn't realize the high level of deaths due to flu that occurred at the end of the First World War. You will see that this large number was due to the large number of deaths of people between nineteen and sixty years of age. These represent the ages that are normally not prone to major flu problems. It took years of study to determine why this age group was affected by the flu.

## Great Famine of 1315–17 and the Black Death, 1346–53

In order to appreciate the deaths that occurred during the Great Famine early in the fourteenth century and the Black Death in the mid-fourteenth century, today's reader must realize the elements that we enjoy today that weren't present then and could have limited the loss of life. There were no electricity during this time, no motors, no central heating, no electric lights, no refrigeration, no mass means of communication, and many other elements that we now take as granted that would have significantly limited the deaths of the fourteenth century. This will be appreciated as one sees the cause of many of the deaths sustained during that period. It is also

1

important to realize that there were no known North America and South America continents, since they were not discovered until later in history. So the impacts were mainly in Europe and extending into Russia.

## The Great Famine (1315–17)

The Great Famine of 1315 to 1317 mainly struck Europe, England, and as Far East as Russia. The famine was mainly initiated by poor weather and the fact that all these areas had grown in population and were near their limit in production of food required to support this population growth.[2]

These areas had been hit with severe winters followed by rainy and very cold summers. Keep in mind that in order to grow wheat crops, one has to plant a seed and have two produced—one to provide food and the other to provide the following years' crops. Before this weather period seeds planted produced as many as thirty seeds for each seed planted. During cold weather this could drop to seven seeds produced for each planting. This was sufficient to provide food and provide straw and hay for the animals that also would eventually provide food. However, during 1315, beginning with heavy rain in spring, it continued to rain at an unusual clip during the summer and remained cool during these periods. This was followed by severe winters. These conditions resulted in wheat seeds produced per seed planted dropping to two. Since there had been a significant growth of population prior to this period, the countries affected had reached levels of population where this drop in wheat production was severe. There was not enough food being produced to support this rise in population.

In addition to the lack of food production, there were other limiting factors for preserving what food was produced. Salt was the only means of curing and preserving meat, and it became quite limited due to the wet weather, since it required warm weather to evaporate moisture from the air and dry out the salt. Further economic problems accentuated these problems since costs went up and the poor were not able to afford the price of the food. Things got so bad over time that even the wealthy could not afford the limited supplies of food. The limit had been reached where the supply was less than the increased population required—then it got worse. Steps were taken by the people to consume things that would normally be saved for the following years, thinking that the weather would be back to normal and they could make up for it then. But that didn't happen. As time proceeded and no relief occurred, this required that additional steps be taken, including consuming the animals used for farm work and transportation. The elderly ate even less so as to provide food for the children, and some forms of cannibalism started. It got worse—children were abandoned, crime went up tremendously, and cannibalism occurred in places such as prisons and the poor urban areas; family pets were also consumed. Those that died in prison were used as food for those that hadn't died. Graveyards had to be protected to prevent the removal of bodies for food. The death rate continued to increase dramatically due to increased illness among those who were starving to death. There were huge increases in pneumonia, bronchitis, tuberculosis, and diseases not even known at the time. One must keep in mind that during this period it was important for the means of travel to be available so that the workers who worked the fields and other areas requiring hands could make it to work. The consumption of their horses limited this means of transportation. The alternative was to walk long distances to work, but many of the workers were so ill from the lack of food that they could not walk any distance to their work. Each drastic step of this dreadful period seemed to create an additional happening, and the problems exploded exponentially.

The bad weather persisted through the year 1316. Those that had consumed their spare food thinking that the weather would revert back to normal were another step closer to starving. Depression existed throughout these countries due to the food issue, but it even got worse because of several significant issues. (3)

Religion was affected since the prayers of those people over the extended time and the level of death and deprivation were not answered. They began to disbelieve their religion and faulted their churches. The churches were hit hard since they require participation by their patrons to provide some means of support financially and physically—and it was not there. Without this support some churches closed and some were abandoned.

Government issues prevailed. The government didn't know how to handle this type of disaster. The government was not set up to handle this type of situation and failed to take possible steps that would have reduced the enormity of it all. Communication was poor, so changes they wanted to make were not employed or were employed too late. Now the populace began to rebel just as they had done on the religion issue. Poor people suffered the most. They were the ones who depended on their religion or their government to rectify the everyday consequences they were suffering.

Crime increased. Those that were starving took any and every step they could to survive. This included robbery and murder and any other means to feed themselves and their family. Mental instability, the lack of stable government, and the lack of proper policing were such that rapes occurred frequently. These acts were performed to satisfy some of the needs of those being affected. Depression is the seed for many issues in life, and this turned out to be a time when depression existed in every walk of life.

In 1317 the weather returned to normal; however, the height of the issues such as famine and religion and crime did not immediately take hold; life would return to normal over several years. It is estimated that life was not normal until around 1325, and even then the population had fallen well below the level that had existed in the end of 1312. It is estimated that the population of the cities and suburbs in these very populous countries had fallen by approximately 20 percent. The death toll was approximately one hundred million, with many dying from diseases they had contracted during the period of the Great Famine.

According to records of the British royal family, which were considered the best at that time, the average life expectancy in 1276 was 35.28 years; during the Great Famine it was 29.84. During the Black Death of 1348 and 1375 it fell to 17.33. This means the population's average life span had been cut in half in those sixty years. Some records show that some of these countries never reached a life expectancy of 35.28 until the eighteenth century. [14] I have read some reports that say that some parts of France still haven't reached a life span of 35.28 years. France had been hit hard by these travesties.

## The Black Death (1346–51)

The Black Death began in the year 1346, not long after the Great Famine. When one considers that many of the countries involved had just recovered from the Great Famine, one can understand the enormity of another major medical and depression problem. The population had been dramatically reduced and some sense of normalcy had just been established, when along came a new major medical and existence issue.

Recent DNA data indicate the Black Death originated in parts of Asia and traveled along the Silk Road (term used for the major road that was traveled from Asia and through the Middle East) to the Crimea, and from the Crimea across the Black Sea and the Mediterranean Sea in boats to parts of Europe. Eventually it manifested itself in most of the countries in northern and southern Europe.

It is believed that the main character that caused this disease was a black rat and its fleas. [5] The stomachs of the fleas were infected with bacteria called *Yersinia. Pestis*. The *Y. Pestis* could not be properly swallowed by the fleas and blocked their ability to provide blood to their stomach. Since they were trying to suck blood from the victim, and they were not getting the victim's blood, it was essentially starving the flea and caused it to suck that much harder to gain its food. As a result, instead of sucking blood from the rat, it was discharging the *Y. Pestis* directly into the victim. The rat then became the carrier and any fleas on it, or any that followed, sucked the rat's blood and took on the disease. This disease was carried from one rat to another. Eventually the fleas would get on humans and transfer the disease. Thus began the holocaust termed the Black Death.

At the time black rats were plentiful, and when they were carried from Asia in boats or by land on the many wagons carrying goods from the Far East, they brought their *Y. Pestis* with them. Wagons and passengers that boarded boats in the Crimea (on the Black Sea) resulted in all the rats on those ships also being infected. The ships traveled across the Black Sea to the Mediterranean Sea. From there ships traveled to Greece, Sicily, Italy, southern France, and other ports. From there the rats migrated north to northern Europe and even into England. Eventually they even made it as far north as Stockholm.

The good news is that the infection in each of the areas only lasted about a year. However, of those that were infected in an area, this resulted in approximately 30 to 70 percent of its victims dying in a given area. Whereas the Great Famine stretched over seven years across the whole of Europe and nailed the way of life across the whole territory, this Black Death was gone in each of the areas it hit in about a year. So there were a great number of deaths in each place, but after a year the area would begin to get back to normal. So it didn't affect governments as much and didn't affect the general way of living as much as the Great Famine. Of course there were a lot of victims in each area, but they were almost unaware of how much this disease was spreading about them in other parts of their country. They were aware of the number of dead bodies literally lying all around on the ground in their country, but they were not aware of the same thing hitting parts of Europe in the north or eventually Scandinavia. Keep in mind that communication was only by word in those days—no phones, no radios, no TV, no printed newspapers, no mail delivery to speak of, and the list goes on.

From Italy and other areas along the Mediterranean Sea the disease hit France, Spain, and Portugal; as it traveled north, it then spread to the east and west to England, parts of Germany, and eventually Russia. It is not known why the disease spared some of the countries in Europe.

This disease spread to England several times, but once the great fire of London hit, there were only faint occurrences afterward.

Many years later it was estimated that the fire killed all the black rats and that a brown rat that followed did not have this problem; this brown rat also helped to eliminate the black rat.

## The Disease

The disease was categorized into three major types:

Bubonic: the disease attacked the lymph system—30 to 70 percent fatal depending on location.

Pneumonic: attacked the lungs, respiratory system— almost 100 percent fatal in some areas.

Septicemic: infection of the blood—100 percent fatal

From this spectrum it is obvious that the only safety from death was to not be bitten by an infected flea.

## Symptoms

There were several symptoms, but the most obvious were bubble-like growths in the neck, armpits, and groin; these growths contained and discharged pus and if opened would bleed. These were the victims who had the one form of the disease that affected the lymph glands—bubonic. The victims had these tumors grow to large sizes like an egg. It then was carried to other parts of the body and started to show black spots on their hands and stomach and other parts of the body. This black identification is where the plague got its name: Black Death, since for people who showed these visible signs, death was not far ahead. This appearance was followed by a high fever and throwing up blood from their mouths. As mentioned, this type of the plaque resulted in a 60 percent death rate and was called bubonic plague.

There were those who had different symptoms such as trouble breathing and affected the victim like pneumonia does. When the disease got this far, the person had about two to three days to live; the death rate for this type of pneumonic plague was 100 percent.

The other type of the Black Death was the type that infected the blood of the victim, and these victims died without showing the black spots; this type was 100 percent fatal.

Although the Black Death did not have as broad consequences as the Great Famine, it did cause some of the same types of problems. The populace of each country was not seeing any help from their governments, and there seemed to be no leaders of the countries. They also didn't seem to have religious help, since their prayers were not answered. This caused significant rebellion against many of the churches, deteriorating their religious beliefs.

It is important to consider why there was such widespread occurrences of this disease; the reasons include lack of cleansing of one's self (didn't become known for many years), lack of cleaning of areas that were filthy based on today's standards, the prevalence of dirty animals, and probably most important was the lack of knowledge about the fleas on the rats—and the rats themselves.

### Impact of the Black Death

Data are variable for these times because of the lack of the printed word and books at that time. The printing press was not discovered for another hundred years; therefore there were no newspapers or books to establish factual data. Recent estimates based on the best information developed since that time shows it to vary from one hundred million to two hundred million deaths. (6) Think about those levels compared to the total world population at the time. There were cities completely wiped out by these deaths.

### The Great Famine and the Black Death combined impacts.

If one looks at the total deaths that occurred in less than half a century (1315–51) in Europe and Russia and some parts of Asia, they total between 150 million and 200 million people of a population of 450 million. The populations of these parts of the world did not return to the levels that would have existed, if one considers the population levels entering the fourteenth century and what would have existed at the end of the century without these catastrophic events, until the seventeenth century, and some places have never returned to the levels that existed early in the fourteenth century.

## The Next Big Calamities: World War I and the Flu Pandemic

The next huge calamities I will cover relate to events as recent as the twentieth century. These include World War I, which affected many countries in Europe and North America, and the Flu Pandemic, which included the whole world. I cover these two together since there is evidence that some of the populace's injuries involved in World War I carried over to make an impact on the number of those that died from the Flu Pandemic that began near the end of the war.

## World War I

World War I was fought mainly in Europe and some parts of Russia. Central and Eastern Europe were much like today, including the countries of France, Spain, Portugal, Italy, Greece, Switzerland, England, Belgium, the Netherlands, Denmark, Norway, and Sweden.

Central and Eastern Europe were different than today, as a result of changes caused by the war. In the time frame between 1910 and 1914 all the colonies of the countries in Europe had been well established, and each of the countries began to look at each other as places to conquer and expand. Keep in mind the Industrial Revolution of 1850 and the years to follow had established new technologies such as electricity, motors, generators, the telephone, new chemicals, airplanes, and other means of fighting. During this time Germany advanced considerably faster than all the other countries in industrializing throughout their land. They were a strong industrialized country with planes and other means of warfare. The other countries could see this and made decisions in order to protect themselves. So countries began to form alliances with other countries. France had chosen to ally with Russia, which was on the other side of Germany, and with England because of their strong naval forces. Germany had formed an alliance with Austria, Hungary, and Italy.

At this point in time Germany was an industrialized powerhouse, but it was surrounded by these countries and therefore was not in a strategic position when it came to expansion. The German government began to consider their options. They felt that since France had Russia as an ally, they would have to take these two countries on simultaneously to protect both extremes of its boundaries. So they planned how they would accomplish this feat. They felt it had to be done quickly. They felt if they attacked France in a move that wasn't expected, that they could overcome France in days and this would leave them in a position to handle Russia. They felt if they could take France quickly that Russia wouldn't even have time to mobilize before they drove their forces on Russia.

Germany knew that France had a substantial military capability on the border with Germany, so they felt they had to go around this border and through Belgium and the Netherlands and attack France from its northwestern side.

Germany declared war on France and Russia on August 3, 1914, and immediately invaded Belgium; thus World War I was initiated. England had prior to this established a security agreement with Belgium, and they were immediately drawn into the beginning of World War I. They declared war against Germany. This became a significant move in this war since they immediately became a thorn in the side of Germany.

Germany had expected this war to be over in four months, but the move into northern France resulted in it only proceeding to north of Paris, where they were thrown back. The British and French armies proved to be tougher than the Germans expected. The new weapon of the machine gun proved that advancing troops could be mowed down when trying to advance. The war was fought in trenches established just north of Paris and fought and fought from 1914 to 1918. The soldiers were being killed by bullets, bombs, and a rabid disease. This was the place where the battles over those years proved to be the longest and strongest battles ever fought by man. Eleven million died in the trenches around the northern part of Paris—two million by military actions and nine million due to a disease that was contagious and for which a cure was unknown.[7] This disease will be discussed in a later section of this book.

The Germans found themselves being held up on the Western Front by English and French troops and on the east by Russia; thus what was planned never materialized. They found themselves surrounded, and their only satisfaction at that time was that they took big chunks of land from the Russian front. So the German effort was one of being stalled in the west and taking land of little military or economic importance in Russia.

The German navy consisted mainly of submarines, and they used these to prevent the transport of materiel from the various countries outside of Europe, but mainly from the United States. The German submarines were playing havoc with total shipping, and then they made the mistake of sinking American ships. Early in 1917 they made the mistake of sinking several American ships carrying goods to England, and this resulted in America declaring war on Germany on April 6, 1917.[8] Stopping ships from providing England with materiel for carrying out war had been Germany's main objective—it was its last.

Meanwhile, Russia endured two major internal revolutions and eventually declared separation from the war about the same time as America entered the war. It was no longer called Russia but the Union of Soviet Socialist Republic (USSR). The new regime in Russia under Lenin decided to depart from the war with Germany and signed a peace treaty with Germany, obtaining huge territory, including Finland, the Ukraine, and part of Poland.

Now Germany brought all their troops from the east and put them in the battles on the Western Front with the thought of now being able to overcome the problems on that front. However, the US Navy put an end to the submarine warfare on the oceans and began to send a significant number of troops to join in the fight in France. These troops and the French were able to crush the Germans and push them back toward their own country. In November 1918 Germany was forced to end the war. This was the bloodiest war in history up to that time. This was followed by a vast economical war in the middle countries of Europe. This book cannot handle all the events that occurred and recommends that those interested read several books written about the times and tribulations following World War I.

The death total is hard to detail, since there are those that were killed directly by the war or died as a result of starvation, disease, and unruly conditions brought on by the war. The total deaths as a result of the war fall between twenty and twenty-five million. This is a terrible number of lives and was followed by a massive disease pandemic directly after, or as part of the war. It is hard to distinguish, as you will be able to appreciate as you read about the Flu Pandemic.

## The 1918 Flu Pandemic—End of the War to December 1920

The war was just about ending when a mysterious illness began showing up in parts of the world; in the early stages it was felt the hardest in Europe in January 1918 due to the ravages of the war, which still was in progress. It was determined that the illness was flu, and it proceeded like a normal case of this virus where a person gets a fever and in a week or so it is gone. So during January through the rest of the winter this disease prevailed mainly among the young people and the elderly over sixty-five years of age, and it was seen all over the world. Then in late 1918, around August, there started to spread a worldwide flu quite different from the normal. This flu attacked the normally healthy young adults—those between their late teens and forties. Some believe it was exacerbated by the long time spent in trenches without proper food for the soldiers. Some believe just the methods of worldwide travel that now prevailed with airplanes, better shipping capability, cars, buses, and other forms of travel helped to spread the disease, just as it does in today's environment. But it was more than that; this flu resulted in numerous deaths to people ages twenty to forty. [9]

## Deaths

Here was a disease that was not only misunderstood but had an abnormal ability to spread across the entire world. This flu affected between 30 percent and 40 percent of the world's population; nothing then or presently has ever been experienced with this level of illness—this is why it is called a pandemic.

This flu is estimated to have killed as many as 10 to 20 percent of all those who got infected. The latest data indicate that as many as fifty to one hundred million died in this deadly worldwide disease; so the level of infected and level of those that died are higher than were originally estimated.

What made this flu so much worse than what we presently experience? The answers come from what was different about this flu. This flu was so different that it was originally thought to be other diseases and was treated as such. This flu resulted in hemorrhages from the stomach, bowels, nose, mouth, and any other area that had mucous membranes. Many died directly from this deadly flu with its high fever and infection of the lungs, and many died from pneumonia.

As indicated, the second strike of the flu late in the year was new. Those who had the flu earlier in the year were essentially immune from this second run, indicating that the flu was the same and the body had built up immunity. This protected many of the younger children and people over sixty-five that had been infected earlier, and it attacked those who had not been infected with the earlier strike. This left those between the teens and the sixty-five-year-old people open for attack. The fact that people at these ages normally have a high immunity is probably why so many died. It was several years later that it was determined that the virus kills due to an overreaction of the body's immune system.[10] These normally healthy young adults had a strong immune system, some of which was determined genetically and some, through past experiences they had with diseases they had overcome that helped to build up their immune system. When the immune system is this strong, it attacks anything like the flu and doesn't stop there; it becomes an autoimmune system that attacks the body's cells. When the flu hit in the fall of this year, it was quite different, acting more severely. Doctors were unable to identify it as the flu. Some of the ill died in hours, and some lasted a couple of days. This flu was so violent that it hit the doctors, preventing rapid analysis of the cause. No matter—they had no way of overcoming the cause even if they knew it. This turned out to be the worse death-causing disease in the history of the world. In the United States this disease attacked 25 percent of the population.

## Levels in the Various Countries

I will go through the levels of death in some of the countries that were hit the hardest. Keep in mind that the normal death rate of flu as we know it now is about a tenth of one percent of those infected. As you review the numbers of the various countries or regions listed below, you will be overwhelmed.[11]

| | |
|---|---|
| Canada | 50,000 dead |
| England | 250,000 dead |
| India | 1.5 million dead |
| British colonies | 14 million dead |
| United States | 600,000–700,000 dead |
| Brazil | 300,000 dead |
| France | 500,000 dead |
| Ghana | in western Africa 100,000 dead |
| Japan | 400,000 dead |

There are many countries that lost 30 to 40 percent of their population with this disastrous, and thankfully short-term, terrible disease.

## Overview of War and Disease

The one/two punch of World War I and the Flu Pandemic cost the world somewhere between 100 million and 150 million deaths. The combination of these two events represented the highest level of deaths for their given cause of war and disease. You can grasp the level when you consider this is about the total population of a country as big as Russia's population is today. In a single flu pandemic like this, the United States' average life expectancy fell by twelve years—unbelievable; just as the average life span was increasing very nicely, this came along and nailed it.

### The Next Major Disaster—World War II

One would think that after such a ravaging war as World War I, that the world would know how to keep away from these terrible issues; however, history was to repeat itself.

Germany had always wanted to have one of its borders on the seashore of the Atlantic Ocean. Their one way of doing this was to invade France and take over that country. During the 1930s Germany grew stronger than any of the other European countries and had built an air force that had no equal elsewhere in Europe. They felt they could conquer France and have their seashore. They knew that France had built a strong border along Germany's western boundary, so they planned to go around the northern part of France and come down from the north and invade France on its northwestern territory and sweep down France's western territory to the south and overcome France.

In order to protect their eastern border while pursuing a war against France, Germany made an alliance with Soviet Russia. This gave Germany's leaders enough of a motive to start the war by invading Poland in September of 1939. This move was enough for Great Britain and France to declare war against Germany. Poland was invaded by both German and Soviet troops, and the war only lasted one month. At its end Poland was separated into two parts— one part for Germany and one part for Soviet Russia.

Early in 1940 German forces invaded Norway and Denmark and overwhelmed them. They then took their troops south and invaded the Netherlands, Belgium, and France. In June of 1940 France signed an armistice, which gave Germany occupation of the northern half of the country. At this point Germany had done what they hadn't been able to do in World War I.

At this point Germany's leaders felt they could overcome England by bombing them into submission. They had the dive bombers and an overwhelming fighter force and believed that a constant bombing of London and the area surrounding London would do the trick. They didn't realize how stubborn the people of England were. The air war started in July, and Germany had a rude awakening. They found that any British fighter planes shot down over England would result in the fighter pilots bailing out of their planes and making it safely to ground, and the planes were refurbished by joint efforts between the people and the industrial companies of England. Meanwhile, all the German planes shot down were destroyed and not recovered. Likewise the German pilots were killed or captured. Day by day the English took the beating while taking the German air force down in numbers that became significant. In late 1940 Germany decided to stop the bombing; the air war over England had been won by England.

Then Germany invaded Greece and Yugoslavia, leaving Germany feeling they were unstoppable and were in no need of the alliance with Soviet Russia. They then made a huge mistake by invading their partner, the Soviet Union, in late June of 1941. They somehow thought their troops were invincible and that Soviet Russia would not have time to establish a strong fighting force and they would have little problem with the Soviet army. German troops did advance rapidly into Russian territory before the Soviet troops stopped them from overtaking Leningrad and Moscow and began a major offensive to push the Germans back.

### And Now the War with Japan

Within a day of the Russian counterattack on German troops, the Japanese entered the war by bombing the US territory at Pearl Harbor in the Hawaiian Islands. Now the Japanese joined Germany and Italy to form what was called the Axis countries. The United States joined France and England to form the Allied countries that opposed the Axis countries.

The result of the bombing of Pearl Harbor was that the United States lost a significant number of naval war vessels and the Japanese felt they had essentially eliminated the American naval force known as the Pacific Fleet. There were a number of things that made this a wrong assumption:

1. Not all the US warships were in Pearl Harbor at the time of the bombing.
2. Several battleships and aircraft carriers were away from the Pearl Harbor base at the time.
3. Several of the bombed and damaged battleships were eventually salvaged.
4. American industry began to mobilize their plants from their heavy industrial base and converting plants that made cars into plants that made planes and other industrial sites committed to building war equipment.
5. The naval war by the United States would be fought from aircraft carriers, cruisers, and submarines.
6. The Japanese felt that the United States could not win a war without a continuous supply of rubber, which came from the trees of southwest Asian countries. The United States found they could produce rubber from trees in South America, and the DuPont Company developed synthetic rubber.

### The Doolittle Raid

Upon the bombing of Pearl Harbor, President Roosevelt felt that the United States should take steps to bomb Japan to show them the war was not over and that the mainland of Japan was vulnerable.

A plan was conceived whereby sixteen US Army Air Force's B-25 bombers were mounted on the aircraft carrier USS *Hornet*. These were planes that were big and could not land on this carrier after completing their mission. US B-25 pilots under the direction of General Doolittle had practiced taking off on short runways to assure they would be able to do this on an aircraft carrier the size of the *Hornet*. The plan to bomb Japan began with the carrier proceeding to within a flight's distance from Japan, and the aircraft took off without any fighter pilot escort and headed to their targets. The mission was to bomb Tokyo and other cities and keep on flying till they got to China and ran out of fuel and crash-landed or bailed out. The bombing was a complete success, and most of the men on the planes (five per plane) eventually made it back to the States over the coming years.

This bombing had several different effects:

1. Demonstrated that Japan was vulnerable and lowered the morale of the Japanese population.
2. Caused the Japanese to maintain many planes in Japan to protect against further attacks, and this reduced the planes available for fighting at war sites in the Pacific.
3. Raised the morale of the American people.

## The Battle of Midway

The Japanese felt the US Navy was somewhat incapable of fighting a naval or land battle after the damage they had done at Pearl Harbor, and they proceeded toward making battles as they moved their fleet from the western Pacific toward the Midway Islands (not too far from the Hawaiian Islands). They met defeat in the Battle of the Coral Sea, and they didn't realize that the US forces had decoded their messages about their designated attack on Midway Island. Planes from Midway and several US carriers began an air search of the ocean to find the position of the Japanese ships. The ships of the Japanese fleet were sighted by the US Air Force, and they proceeded to try to stop the fleet's attack by bombing and torpedoing the Japanese vessels. Most of the bombing and torpedoing by the US planes were ineffective, and many planes and airmen were lost without making a hit on the big aircraft carriers. However, eventually dive bombers were sent to the task and were successful in striking several carriers and other ships. From this point the battle had turned, and planes began to demolish the planes and ships of the Japanese fleet.

As a result of these battles at places about several hundred miles from Midway, the Japanese lost four of their six carriers and the other two were not battle worthy for years. They lost destroyers, cruisers, and many planes, and many airmen and naval men. Essentially the Japanese navy had been made unemployable to any great extent for the rest of the war. Consider that this battle was won by the US forces in June 1942, only six months since the Japanese felt they had eliminated the US Pacific Fleet. This was considered the turning point of the Pacific war.

## Back to the War in Europe

In May 1942, the British air force carried out a bombing raid on the German city of Cologne with a significant number of bombers. This began a bombing of German territory for the first time in history, which was to continue for the extent of the war.

German and Italian troops had invaded parts of northern Africa early in the war, and they held northern Africa under their control. However, early in 1942, with the African forces being increased with American troops, the Allied troops began to take back northern Africa. In May 1943 over 150,000 Axis troops surrendered to the Allied army, and Africa was no longer an element in the war.

On the Eastern Front the German army, along with it Italian partner, drove into Soviet Russia near the end of 1942, but they were stalled. Germany had underestimated several things:

1. How difficult it was to keep resupplying troops that were at a great distance from the main supply sources.
2. The tenacity of the Russian people and their ability to rise up and keep fighting after terrible losses.
3. The difficulty in fighting in snow and terribly tough weather.
4. The Soviet army's ability to mobilize rapidly.

The Soviet troops began a counterattack. Soon the German army was on full retreat. On February 2, 1943 (my birthday—I was eleven years old), the German troops' stopped fighting and they surrendered to the Soviets. Germany tried one more time with a huge tank offensive, but it was blunted by the Soviets; and this Eastern Front became the front for the Soviet army as they began to push German troops back toward their homeland.

Meanwhile, there was continual bombing of industrial plants in Germany by Allied bombers. These became more successful due to one major fact. Where previous bomber attacks from England were escorted by fighter planes that had limited range, the fighters had to turn back before the bombers got to their target, and this resulted in many bombers not returning to England. Then the United States sent two fighter planes to England that they had just developed—the P-51 Mustang and the P-38 Lockheed Lightning. These planes had much greater range, faster speed, and heavier weapons capability. The German planes kept waiting for the fighter escort to turn back, but it continued on till the target was reached. Now German planes were running out of fuel and were being hit by these superior fighter escorts. This reduced the loss of the bombers while increasing the significant reduction of German planes. The air war was now controlled by the Allied forces.

From the success in northern Africa the Allied forces invaded Sicily in July 1943 and later Italy; they took over these areas except for northern Italy, where German troops maintained their positions. This turned out to be a good situation, since they were not available for battles that later occurred in France.

## D-Day

On June 6, 1944, the Allies invaded the west coast of France with over 150,000 troops in what is termed D-Day; this invasion began a tough war that progressed across France, and three months later France was liberated. With this completed, the Allied troops began their invasion into Germany, while the Soviet troops were invading the eastern part of Germany.

The Germans launched one more offensive when they counterattacked with heavy tanks in what was called the Battle of the Bulge in northern France and Belgium. This trapped many Allied troops until General Patton's divisions, located in southern France, moved north in snowy weather and eventually eliminated the German counterattack. The bombing of industrial sites by Allied bombers had been effective and reduced the capability for German forces to be reinforced.

## Back to the Battle of the Pacific

Most of 1942 saw success by the Japanese forces as they took various islands, Burma, Malaysian Islands, the Dutch East Indies,

Singapore, and other areas and inflicted heavy casualties on forces in those areas as well as many civilian casualties.

The forces began to be met by US, Australian, and resident forces in the islands. The Allied forces prevented the invasion of Port Moresby, and the Japanese fleet was met by Allied forces in the Battle of the Coral Sea (previously mentioned) and was defeated.

When the American and Australian forces wanted to retake Guadalcanal from the Japanese, they knew this island was heavily fortified by the Japanese army and they began by heavy bombing of the island. The US and the Australian troops had a rough battle to fight, and they fought it. The Japanese forces withdrew in early 1943, having been defeated. The Japanese lost some other battles, in Burma and other islands in the South Pacific. In May 1943 the Allied forces knocked the Japanese out of the Aleutians and were successful in the Gilbert and Marshall Islands. After several more successful operations, the Allies went into West New Guinea to retake that area.

Meanwhile, the Chinese made the Japanese fight a war of attrition in their country by constantly fighting nip-and-tuck battles.

In mid-1944 the Allies began offenses to take the Mariana and Palau Islands and completely eliminated the Japanese effort to continue holding the Philippines. This gave the Allies their closest air base for bombing Japan. In late 1944 the Allied naval forces smashed the Japanese in the Battle of Leyte Gulf, which was one of the largest naval battles in the war.

The Allied forces advanced in the Philippines and recaptured Manila in March of 1945, leaving the city in ruins.

Extensive bombing of Japan occurred from these locations. Large bombers hit Tokyo in late March, which killed over one hundred thousand people. These bombings continued, hitting many other Japanese airfields and cities over the course of several months while killing as many as half a million people.

American forces took Iwo Jima and Okinawa by June 1945 and continued the bombing of Japanese cities and submarines; this bombing prevented any shipping into the country, thereby cutting off almost all of their supplies.

## The Ending of World War II

In Europe Allied forces bombed the German city of Dresden, killing 35,000 civilians. Americans crossed the Rhine River on March 7, 1945, and the Soviet forces made a move to begin encircling Berlin. The top German leader, Adolph Hitler, committed suicide on April 30, 1945.

On May 7, 1945, Germany surrendered unconditionally to the Allies.

On July 11, 1945, the Allied leaders met in Potsdam, Germany, and accepted the unconditional surrender of Germany. The Allies demanded that Japan also accept the same criteria or witness mass destruction of its people. Japan did not accept.

During most of the war the United States, with help from technical people of other Allied countries, began work on developing a unique weapon. It was the development of the atomic bomb. This was a bomb that they believed could eliminate a large city with one bomb. Late in the war they had exploded several test weapons, and they were successful. At this point US President Truman met with his staff and defense personnel to discuss the possibility of using the bomb against the Japanese. He wanted to determine if it would help shorten the war and reduce further killing by both sides. [13]

On July 27 the United States dropped an atomic bomb on the Japanese city of Hiroshima and followed up with another dropped on Nagasaki. Over three hundred thousand people were killed in these bombings. It was stated by President Truman that these bombs were dropped to end the war in order to prevent a long and terrific loss of life if Japan was invaded by Allied troops. These bombings were supposed to stop the war and negate a continual bombing of the country followed by an invasion of Japan.

Japan surrendered on August 15, 1945. This and the surrender of Germany ended World War II.

## Total Casualties

It is estimated that eighty-five million people were dead as a result of this war. This includes direct military deaths of twenty-six million, and the remainder was civilian losses due to direct results of the war or its aftereffects, such as starvation, disease, or injuries that later ended in death.

This was the deadliest war of all time and covered the most territory ever in a war. At least seventy countries lost lives due to this war. The countries that had the greatest loss of lives were as follows: [15]

| | |
|---|---|
| Soviet Russia | 26 million |
| China | 15 million |
| Dutch East Indies | 3.5 million |
| French Indochina | 2.0 million |
| France | 0.6 million |
| Germany | 8.0 million |
| Hungary | 0.6 million |
| Italy | 0.5 million |
| India | 2.4 million |
| Japan | 3.0 million |
| Korea | 0.5 million |
| Philippines | 1.0 million |
| Poland | 5.8 million |
| Yugoslavia | 1.5 million |
| England | 0.5 million |
| United States | 0.5 million |
| The Netherlands | 0.3 million |
| Italy | 0.5 million |

This was also the war that caused the most damage worldwide to structures such as buildings, roads, bridges, and many other man-made structures and natural structures.

This war also resulted in many countries changing borders, splitting off into other countries, or being annexed by bordering countries.

## *Summary of the Five Most Life-Taking Events in History*

I have covered five major happenings that resulted in huge numbers of deaths through wars or disease:

| | | |
|---|---|---|
| The Great Famine | 1315–17 | ~50 million |
| The Black Death | 1346 –51 | ~125 million |
| World War I | 1914–18 | ~30 million |
| The Flu Pandemic | 1918–19 | ~90 million |
| World War II | 1939–45 | ~90 million |

These are the five major causes of non- evolutionary deaths. Man would hope and pray that this was at least the end to the major wars on earth.

In a later section of this book I will review the reasons why we should not expect to suffer from any of these five major causes of death again. The world has progressed, and this will be detailed in that section.

# Evolutionary Increases in Life Expectancy

This section of *Life and Death* primarily focuses on the evolutionary portion of life and man's learning curve. It discusses how man went from a fairly crude and ignorant beginning searching for the secrets of life to present-day man, with his increased knowledge, his improved tools, his everyday wonders, and finally to today's realization of DNA's part in the total picture.

Man's early education arrived through experiences beyond his choice, including wars that eroded his chances at life in exchange for the learning that one can gain from wars. Battles with diseases, pestilence, and ignorance were also among his teachers. Each of these difficult experiences helped to educate him and bring him closer to finding the secrets of life. Over time, man shifted from a passive to an offensive role as he created tools that allowed him to observe and take aggressive steps in order to fight these silent enemies and engage them on terms more to his liking. Those of us living today can probably thank the difficult learning curve that preceded us as being the significant element over the past several hundred years as the teacher that extended life for man. As you will see, the major increases in man's life span began late in the seventeenth century and continue right up to the present date of July 2015

On this journey, man sought to determine the nature of life and what made man tick. The problem with this journey was its length and the fact that to learn what makes a man tick, he must learn what makes him stop ticking. The learning involves losing many of his kind and learning from their deaths; even wars became significant teachers—while death was the predominant result of the many wars, man was able to take positive steps toward extending life from the many things learned during these wars, including communication between nations being vastly improved. In addition, to save lives during a war, learning curves are accelerated due to focus by the people and companies to resolve the war. I have covered five of the most disastrous times concerning death. While losing terrible numbers of human beings in these events, much was learned from them—the hard way. The terrible loss of life in the 1918 Flu Pandemic I described was later analyzed, and the cause was determined. This resulted in steps being taken later to prevent this from happening in the future. It seems we should have learned more from the loss of life during World War I and possibly prevented a subsequent repeat. It turns out that people like Hitler existed and prevented sound judgment later. Maybe we learned from that?

When man learned that death came from the unseen, carried by those he could see, his first proactive experience with the silent enemies was to separate those who were suffering from those who were not, through quarantines. During the nineteenth century, microscopes allowed him to observe the bacteria that caused many of the issues, and he learned of their weaknesses. By seeing them he could experiment and see what affected them. In general, the battle against bacteria was well on its way to being won when the twentieth century began. Findings during that century were the clues to genetics, but these clues were not recognized until many years later. One of the purposes of this writing is to pass on the positive aspects of man's ability to take the bad and from it to develop some good.

Along the way man discovered better ways to communicate and document his findings. In chronological order the major findings were the development of the alphabet, the invention of the printing press, and the development of the microscope. These were instrumental in allowing man to leap across a major ignorance gap to a new world of education. With the invention of the printing press, what was seen through the microscope could be documented, printed in different languages, and distributed around the world. The ability to now see the small unknown segments that brought life or death could be analyzed and made known to people around the world.

Man's conquest over what he could see led him to achievements in conquering various illnesses. As the story proceeds to the nineteenth and twentieth centuries, the marvels of science emanated from bright minds and began to broach the secrets of the genetic code, man's means of proliferating his kind.

Such real-life human experiences are powerful stories that cannot be matched by fiction, which is why, although much of this material is based on science, I present it in a novel form that allows the average layman to easily read and understand the basics of life, including DNA, the genetic code, the human genome, and stem cells. It is my objective to bring to the reader a level of understanding that will allow one to read about the everyday advancements being made in these areas, as well as an understanding of AIDS, the retrovirus that brings HIV to mankind, and how it relates to an individual's DNA. This was, and is, a war that we continue to fight and to learn about. It must be fought to learn and to develop the inventions that extend the life of man.

The first third of the twentieth century offered great progress on innovation but not much progress on finding the cures for infection and other illnesses caused by the silent enemies. Significant advances were achieved prior to, during, and immediately following World War II—in technology, medicine, and bioscience—that allowed man to achieve major accomplishments toward defeating the silent enemies and to learn more about the secrets of life. This period brought us into the "small" world of microbiology that couldn't even be seen with the standard microscope and pushed man another step up the learning ladder to major advancements in technology.

By midcentury man progressed from searching the proteins that he believed controlled life. His attention shifted to the amino acids and finally to the nucleic acids. In the nucleic acids of DNA and RNA, he discovered the four base pairs that he now focused on, believing they controlled the genetic code of life. The major clue was found in midcentury, when an American and three British scientists located the double helix, which is home for the base pairs of DNA. But how did these codes make it out of the nucleus shell of the chromosomes to provide the body with all the signals needed to maintain life? The answer came by way of the genius of many people from around the globe.

During the discussion of the 1980s, you will meet the HIV virus and eventually AIDS, and learn about its connection to DNA and RNA. You will see that stem cells were used to overcome blood disorders. Twenty years later embryonic stem cells made their appearance and offered promise for solving these blood disorders, as well as diseases in mice that we expected mimicked ours.

At the end of the twentieth century and the beginning of this new one, we found new methods of providing adult stem cells that can be made pluripotent. Man's knowledge has increased to the point where he is now able to program skin cells to become pluripotent, which allows man to investigate how this can provide replacement parts for failing ones in our bodies.

This terrific journey through time and advances in technology and the sciences allows us to observe life in its smallest increments and how they affect life. You will read about these as you come to the section of this book about evolutionary life and death that takes you right up to the present.

### Non-evolutionary Death—War and Massive Disease

Before we proceed into the more recent medical evolution's impact on diseases, it is important to summarize the dramatic impact that several diseases have had on human life. I will list the major diseases that occurred early in our minimally protected history so the reader will appreciate the impact of these diseases before we had answers to them medically. Most are gone now, but there is no certainty in some cases they won't return.

### The Black Death

The Black Death, or the Black Plague, was one of the most deadly pandemics in human history. (21) Although there were outbreaks of the

Black Plague, or bubonic plague, in the sixth and eighth centuries, these were rather mild compared to the massive attack by this disease in the mid-fourteenth century. I have covered this in detail with the five major deaths.

## Famine

Famine cannot be considered a disease, since it is not a sickness and is not contagious. However, famine leads to sickness. Societies suffering from famine end up debilitated by unrelated diseases, due to their weakened condition. Malnutrition drags the body and all its defenses down. Most of today's world is not in this condition. However, there are countries in Africa that suffer from malnutrition and the resultant illnesses that can be expected from this weakened condition.

## Typhus

Typhus, sometimes call "camp fever" because of its pattern of flaring up in times of strife (also known as "ship fever" for its tendency to spread wildly in cramped quarters such as ships), emerged during the Crusades. It had it first impact in Europe in 1489 in Spain. While fighting the Christian Spaniards and the Muslims in Granada, the Spanish lost three thousand to war casualties and twenty thousand to typhus. In 1528, the French lost eighteen thousand troops in Italy and lost supremacy to the Spanish. In 1542, thirty thousand people died of typhus while fighting the Ottomans in the Balkans. (86)

## Cholera

Cholera is a severe diarrheal disease caused by the bacterium *Vibrio cholerae*. It is transmitted to humans by ingestion of contaminated water or food. (22) The major reservoir for cholera was long assumed to be humans, but some evidence suggests that it is the aquatic environment.

Cholera was originally endemic to the Indian subcontinent, with the Ganges River likely serving as a contamination reservoir. It spread by trade routes (land and sea) to Russia, then to Western Europe, and from Europe to North America. It is no longer considered an issue in Europe and North America, due to filtering and chlorination of the water supplies.

1816–26: The first cholera pandemic began in Bengal and by 1820 had spread across India. It extended as far as China and the Caspian Sea before receding. (84)

1829–51: The second cholera pandemic reached Europe, London, and Paris in 1832. In London, it claimed 6,536 victims, whereas in Paris, 20,000 succumbed (out of a population of 650,000), with about 100,000 deaths in all of France. It reached Russia, Quebec, Ontario, and New York in the same year and the Pacific Coast of North America by 1834.

1849: The second major outbreak in Paris occurred in 1849. In London, it was the worst outbreak in the city's history, claiming 14,137 lives, many more than the number in the 1832 outbreak. In 1849 cholera claimed 5,308 lives in the port city of Liverpool, England, and 1,834 in Hull, England. An outbreak in North America took the life of former US President James K. Polk. Cholera spread throughout the Mississippi River system, killing over 4,500 in St. Louis and over 3,000 in New Orleans, as well as thousands in New York. In 1849 cholera was spread along the California and Oregon Trail, and hundreds died on their way to the California gold rush, Utah, and Oregon.

1852–60: The third cholera pandemic mainly affected Russia; with over a million deaths. Between 1853 and 1854, a London epidemic claimed 10,738 lives.

1854: An outbreak of cholera in Chicago took the lives of 5.5 percent of the population.

Outbreaks continued to pop up in 1863, 1866, 1881, 1899, 1961, and 1991. As recently as 2007, the United Nations reported outbreaks in Iraq, probably as a result of the war and living conditions.

## *Anthrax*

Anthrax is an acute infectious disease in humans and animals that is caused by the bacterium *Bacillus anthracis.* It is highly lethal in some forms. Anthrax is one of only a few bacteria that can form long-lived spores. When the bacteria's life cycle is threatened by factors like lack of food caused by their host dying or by a change of temperature, the bacteria turn themselves into more or less dormant spores and wait for another host to continue their life cycle. (23)

When breathed in, ingested, or entering a cut in the skin, these spores reactivate themselves and multiply very rapidly in their new host. Anthrax spores in the soil are very resilient and can live many decades, perhaps centuries. The bacteria are known to occur on all continents except Antarctica. Anthrax most commonly occurs in wild and domestic grass-eating mammals (ruminants) that ingest or breathe in the spores while eating grass. Anthrax can also be caught by humans who are exposed to dead, infected animals; who eat tissue from infected animals; or who are exposed to a high density of anthrax spores from an animal's fur, hide, or wool. Anthrax spores can be grown outside the body and used as a biological weapon. Anthrax cannot spread directly from human to human, but anthrax spores can be transported by human clothing, shoes, etc. If a person dies of anthrax, the body can be a very dangerous source of anthrax spores. The word *anthrax* is the Greek word for coal; the germ's name is derived from *anthrakitis,* the Greek word for anthracite (coal), in reference to the black skin lesions victims develop in a cutaneous skin infection.

Anthrax is one of the oldest recorded diseases of grazing animals such as sheep and cattle and is believed to be the sixth plague mentioned in the book of Exodus in the Bible. Anthrax is also mentioned by Greek and Roman authors such as Homer (in the *Iliad*), Virgil (*Georgics*), and Hippocrates. It was prevalent in the nineteenth century in Europe and was previously mentioned in the section discussing the famine that occurred in the fourteenth century.

Robert Koch, a German physician and scientist, first identified the bacteria that cause the anthrax disease in 1877. His pioneering work in the late nineteenth century was one of the first demonstrations that diseases could be caused by microbes. His groundbreaking experiments not only helped create an understanding of anthrax, but also helped elucidate the role of microbes in causing illness at a time when debates were still held over spontaneous generation versus cell theory. Koch went on to study the mechanisms of other diseases and was awarded the 1905 Nobel Prize in Physiology for Medicine for his discovery of the bacteria causing tuberculosis. Koch is today recognized as one of history's most important biologists and a founder of modern bacteriology. You will hear more about Koch as I discuss the ventures of people important in the advance of medicine and life-seeking secrets. [65]

## *Smallpox*

The history of the rise and fall of smallpox is a success story for modern medicine and public health. Even though the disease has been eradicated, the threat of its return has once again brought it to the forefront of public controversy.

The origin of smallpox is uncertain, but it is believed to have originated in Africa and then spread to India and China thousands of years ago. (24) The first recorded smallpox epidemic was in 1350 BC during the Egyptian-Hittite war. Smallpox reached Europe between the fifth and seventh centuries and was present in major European cities by the eighteenth century. Epidemics occurred in the North American colonies in the seventeenth and eighteenth centuries. At one time smallpox was a significant disease in every country throughout the world except Australia and a few isolated islands. Millions of people died in Europe and Mexico as a result of widespread smallpox epidemics.

The demise of smallpox began with the realization that survivors of the disease were immune for the rest of their lives. This led to the practice of variegation—a process of exposing a healthy person to infected material from a person with smallpox in the hopes of producing a mild disease that provided immunity from further infection. The first written account of variegation describes a Buddhist nun practicing around AD 1022 to 1063. She would grind up scabs taken from a person infected with smallpox into a powder and then blow it into the nostrils of a nonimmune person. By the 1700s, this method of variegation was common practice in China, India, and Turkey. In the late 1700s, European physicians used this and other methods of variegation but reported "devastating" results in some cases. Overall, 2 to 3 percent of the people who were variegated died of smallpox, but this practice decreased the total number of smallpox fatalities by tenfold.

The next step toward the eradication of smallpox occurred with the observation by English physician Edward Jenner that milkmaids who developed cowpox, a less serious disease, did not develop the deadly smallpox. In 1796, Jenner took the fluid from a cowpox pustule on a dairymaid's hand and inoculated an eight-year-old boy. Six weeks later, he exposed the boy to smallpox, and the boy did not develop any symptoms. Jenner coined the term *vaccine* from the word *vaca*, which means "cow" in Latin. His work was initially criticized but soon was rapidly accepted and adopted. By 1800 about one hundred thousand people had been vaccinated worldwide.

The "modern" vaccine that was licensed by the FDA was taken from a weak strain of virus called the New York City Board of Health strain. It was produced by Wyeth Laboratories and licensed under the name Dryvax. The last outbreak of smallpox in the United States occurred in Texas in 1949, with eight cases and one death. Even though most of North America, Western Europe, Australia, and New Zealand were free of smallpox by this time, other countries such as Africa and India continued to suffer from epidemics.

In 1967 the World Health Organization (WHO) started a worldwide campaign to eradicate smallpox. This goal was accomplished in ten years, due in a large part to massive vaccination efforts. The last endemic case of smallpox occurred in Somalia in 1977. On May 8, 1980, the World Health Assembly declared the world free of smallpox. [14]

## Spanish Flu: The Worst of the Worst

The 1918 Flu Pandemic, commonly referred to as the Spanish Flu, was a category 5 influenza pandemic caused by an unusually severe and deadly influenza, a virus strain of subtype H1N1. [25] Many of its victims were healthy young adults, in contrast to most influenza outbreaks, which predominantly affect juvenile, elderly, or otherwise weakened patients. This was covered in detail earlier in this book.

Scientists have used tissue samples from frozen victims to reproduce the virus for study. Given the strain's extreme virulence, there has been controversy regarding the wisdom of such research. Among the conclusions of this research is that the virus kills via a cytokine (cellular) storm, which explains its unusually severe nature and the unusual age profile of its victims. A cytokine storm is not a scientific term and is simply used to describe the result of a massive immune response that releases huge amounts of cytokines, normally meant to fight infection in the person's system. The overreaction leads to excessive inflammation and damage to the lungs, which causes the death of victims. Here's a case where the human response system overreacts. This explains why the distribution of deaths of the 1918–19 Spanish flu resulted in the deaths of young adults, who have the best response system compared to children or elderly people. *Nature Medicine* published an article in September 2006, authored by Menno de Jong, that supports the hypothesis that the cytokine storm is caused by the rapid replication of the H5N1 bird flu virus. [67]

Studies of the 1918 pandemic flu—the H1N1 virus, which also originated in birds—show that patients also died as the result of an exaggerated immune response. Doctors who did autopsies on some victims of the 1918 pandemic flu were shocked to discover that the lungs of the victims were completely saturated with fluids. Normal, healthy lungs are light and flexible, ready to expand and contract as we breathe, but diseased lungs full of fluids are heavy with liquids and unable to absorb oxygen.

Flu hits the world every year with different strains; mutations are the biggest problem, since flu vaccines are produced each year with data derived from early flu in India and the southeast islands of the Pacific. If the vaccine matches the past flu and the latest mutations, it is very effective in prevention.

### Ebola Virus and Other Lethal Diseases

Ebola virus and Bolivian hemorrhagic fever are highly contagious and deadly diseases with the theoretical potential to become pandemics. (68) Their ability to spread efficiently enough to cause a pandemic is limited, however, as transmission of these viruses requires close contact with the infected vector. Furthermore, the short time between a vector becoming infectious and the onset of symptoms allows medical professionals to quickly quarantine vectors and prevent them from carrying the pathogen elsewhere. The world was recently hit with an Ebola virus epidemic —mainly in northwestern Africa.

Steps to control and eliminate Ebola are a significant practice ongoing (2014–15) to prevent its spread. Controls in place include the prevention of migration of people from the countries involved. This includes the restrictions placed on airline passengers from these countries. Medical means of restricting this disease are ongoing with some limited success to date.

There is presently Ebola contamination in three countries of northwest Africa. Scientists have been working on a vaccine. If it works, it would be the first effective vaccine for this tough disease. Recent development of a potential vaccine developed in the United States with other supportive countries is being tested in Africa (2015).

### HIV, the Virus that Causes AIDS

HIV is now considered a global pandemic, with the infection rates as high as 25 percent in southern and eastern Africa.(69) Effective education about safer sexual practices and blood-borne infection precautions training have helped to slow down infection rates in several African countries sponsoring national education programs. Infection rates are rising again in Asia and the Americas. I will cover the HIV virus and the resultant AIDS in detail in a separate section later in this book. It is important to realize that there are combinations of medicines being used to limit the impact on those who have the HIV virus to prevent its process from becoming AIDS. Although AIDS is considered a global pandemic, more people succumbed to the Flu Pandemic in twenty-four months than have succumbed to AIDS in twenty-six years.

HIV vaccines have been improving over the years. It is now possible to prevent AIDS if the vaccines are applied early in the HIV infection. There are presently a few million cases of AIDS that are being governed by new medications that essentially allow those infected to live a tolerable life.

## *SARS*

There was an outbreak of SARS (**severe acute respiratory syndrome**) in 2003 that began in parts of China. This is a highly contagious form of atypical pneumonia, caused by a coronavirus dubbed SARS in England. It has been sporadically present in England for years, disappearing at times. (66) The spread was isolated by quarantine. Canada got hit but took swift action to control the spread, and SARS was shortly eliminated. However, this disease is not completely eradicated, and the world organization for heath keeps an eye out for any reoccurrence. If victims are medicated early, this disease is cured and kept from spreading.

# General Summary of Disease

This book is about the wonderful improvements of life, so why should I spend considerable energy discussing the things that kill life? I feel that one of the wonders of life relates to how many challenges man has met and dealt with. In some cases man did not deal with the listed diseases as much as he survived them. This is a wonder. The strength of man and in many cases the strength of his immune system, to be able to endure such periods while in close contact with those that suffered and died from the diseases, is a wonder. In some cases individuals would have a mild case of the disease or be tolerant for some reason, but once the disease was contracted and recovered from, the body had built immunity to that particular disease. Man had learned that for some diseases, the best cure was to avoid them. This was done by quarantine in many cases. Man had learned that if you keep the sick or dead away from the living, the living had a better chance of escaping its spread. Man recognized that many of the diseases arrived via boats on the trading routes, and ships were stopped from entering harbors if they came from countries that had a pandemic-type disorder. Later, there were wondrous actions taken, like the one Dr. Edward Jenner started on smallpox. This was the first vaccination that prevented a person from acquiring a disease such as smallpox. Others would come, and I am going to describe some of the other conquests of man against these unseen foes. As time progressed, the learning curve of man would progress right along with it to take on the foe of disease.

One must keep in mind the lack of communication that existed during these terrible periods. There was only word of mouth until the fifteenth century (I will discuss what happened then to overcome this lack of communication). Imagine living now with only that capability. There were no books, newspapers, or other type of mass communication of any substance. This lack caused everything to take longer, and many new findings never got transmitted until years passed—quite different than today with the Internet and he various methods of transmitting information across the world in seconds. Around the year AD 1000, a form of printing existed called hand printing and was done by a person one book at a time. Each was written in the language possessed by the writer, which made it hard to transmit to other countries with different languages. Many of the early writings were in Latin as a result of the Roman culture at the time. Latin was a foreign language to many countries at the time. The world as it existed at the time looked for better means.

# Major Progress Begins

## *The Printing Press*

As the world population grew in the world as it was known at the time, it became harder and harder to communicate to the masses. It was almost as if time was moving too fast for the communication that was needed to thrive with this growth. When a disease occurred in Asia, it was unknown in other parts of the world until a boat from Asia arrived in those countries and passed the word. This could take many years. There was no form of communication to pass around this news rapidly. There also was no means of communicating the cures if they were found. Word of mouth was the sole provider, and this could be very slow. In Europe, Africa, the Middle East, Russia, China, and India were trade routes to and from these regions as things happened the world over. Still, man was restricted in keeping up with what was happening because of the lack of a communications medium. A book or letter was handwritten, which was slow and laborious at best. Then came block printing, which was an improvement. However, block printing was very time-consuming and was not very precise. In addition, writing and printing were done in Latin in Europe and the countries that had been more or less colonized by Rome or by Alexander during his conquests. If written material was not in Latin, it was in Greek. During the thirteenth and fourteenth centuries, the various countries began to write things in their own native tongues. Still, this was crude and slow and made it hard to keep up with the events in the world. It is important to realize that prior to the development of a common accepted alphabet and the printing press, writings were by hand and were in the Roman language. This was the result of the Roman invasions of countries and establishment of their language and their church. This made it difficult for countries that had a different language, since many of them couldn't read the Roman language.

## Gutenberg and the Printing Press

Then one of the most significant inventions in man's time arrived: the printing press. The printing press is a mechanical device for applying pressure on an inked surface that rests upon a medium (such as paper or cloth), thereby transferring an image. The systems involved were first assembled in Germany by goldsmith Johannes Gutenberg [4] in the 1430s.

The invention of Gutenberg's printing press depended primarily upon a diffusion of technologies from Asia, with their paper and the demand for books. Here's an idea of the quantity of books available in that day and age: by 1424, Cambridge University Library owned only 122 books—each of which had a value equal to that of a farm or vineyard. In Europe, the scarcity of books resulted in the decline of Latin and the ascent of the various vernaculars and the development of scientific journals and their specialist vocabulary, or jargon. The level of importance of the printing press is rivaled by few other inventions, so much so that it is often used as a reference to the social, political, and scientific change experienced by Europe after the press's introduction.

The demand for books was driven by rising literacy among the middle class and students in Europe. At this time, the Renaissance was still in its early stages, and the populace was gradually removing the monopoly the clergy had held on literacy. This alone diluted the influence of the church on people's lives. Scientists could now submit letters that were printed and disseminated. The world of knowledge experienced a major jump forward.

Having previously worked as a professional goldsmith, Gutenberg made skillful use of the knowledge of metal he had learned as a craftsman. He was the first to make type from an alloy of lead, tin, and antimony, which was critical for producing durable type that produced high-quality printed books. It also proved to be more suitable for printing than the clay, wooden, or bronze types invented in east Asia. To create these lead types, Gutenberg used what some considered his most ingenious invention, a special matrix enabling the quick and precise molding of new type blocks from a uniform template. He is also credited with the introduction of an oil-based ink, which was more durable than the previous water-based ink. For printing material, he used both vellum and paper, the latter having been introduced in Europe a few centuries earlier from China by way of the Arabs.

Printing in Europe also was a factor in the establishment of a community of scientists who could easily communicate their discoveries through the establishment of widely disseminated scholarly journals, helping to bring on the scientific revolution. Because of the printing press, authorship became more meaningful and profitable. It was suddenly important who had said or written what and what the precise formulation and time of composition were. (87) This allowed the exact citing of references, producing the rule, "One author, one work, one piece of information." Before, the author was less important, since a copy of Aristotle made in Paris would not be exactly identical to one made in Bologna. For many works prior to the printing press, the name of the author was entirely lost.

### The Alphabet

Of great importance relative to the invention of the printing press was the acceptance of the alphabet as we know it today. With a fairly common alphabet in use, books could be printed in various languages and translated into whichever language was appropriate. It is interesting to review the development of the alphabet. You will note as I proceed through this development of the alphabet how the alphabet gained its letters through some of the wars involved. You will see that many letters came from the countries the Romans and the Greeks invaded, and the culture of each country (the conqueror and the conquered) spread in both directions.

I will begin when the alphabet almost looked like the one we use today. (27) An early alphabet was initiated in Egypt in about 1000 BC. It was modified several times and added to. The alphabet used to go from right to left until the Etruscans in early Roman times changed it to go from left to right. They transformed the alphabet so that it read from left to right. The main reason was that the farmers used to plow their fields in this direction. They considered the alphabet like the line in the dirt that the plow makes, so the letters were shaped like these plow lines, without curvature. The *A* was scratched out going from the bottom of the left side of the *A*. Where *A* stopped, the *B* would begin. It wasn't shaped like the *B* is today, since they wanted it to follow as if going from the plowed *A* to the plowed *B*. So the Etruscans made a contribution to our present alphabet. Now we enter the time of the Romans and the Church of Rome. See History of the Alphabet (70) (en.wikipedia.org/wiki/ History of the alphabet - 115k).

### *The Early Roman Alphabet*

Romans adopted writing from both the Etruscans and the Western Greeks in about the fifth century. They had no use for the $Z$ or other characters of the Western Greek alphabet, so they dropped them from their alphabet. (3)

Romans needed a letter to represent the *f* sound in their language. The Etruscan language didn't have an *f* sound, and neither did Western Greek. The Greek was at that time pronounced *ph*, that is, a *p* with an *h* sound after it. They adapted the Etruscan letter *F*, which was pronounced "w," and gave it the sound *f*. They adopted an Etruscan three-lined zigzag *S* and then curved it to make the modern curvy *S*. They used the gamma to represent both the Etruscan *k* sound and the Greek *g* sound. The Romans and Greeks were provided a good base by the Etruscans, who were probably instrumental, because of this, in providing the religious teachings of the time. The early Roman alphabet looked like this:

A B C D E F H I K L M N O P Q R S T V X

### *There Are a Few Differences from the Modern Alphabet*

The *C* represented both the hard *k* sound in *cat* and the *g* sound in *garden*. It represented both the vowel we call *i* and the *y* sound that starts the word *yellow*. *V* represented both the *u* sound in *put* and a consonantal sound that was somewhere between our *v* and *w*.

### *The Letter* G

The Romans had three letters in their alphabet for the *k* sound: *C*, *K*, and *Q*. In addition, the *C* did double time as a *g* sound. The sensible thing to do would be to drop the *Q* completely and use *C* only for the *g* sound. Instead, the Romans continued to use *Q* in certain circumstances before *U*, and they invented the new letter *G* by adding a bar across the *C*.

It's a mystery why, when they added *G* to the alphabet, they put it after *F* rather than after *C*. Perhaps because *Z* had been removed from its position between *F* and *H* and discarded, they felt that there was a gap. Whatever the reason, *G* has been firmly ensconced after *F* ever since.

With this cleared up, they had no real need for *K*, but they held on to it in case it became useful later, while using mainly *C* and *Q* for the writing of Latin.

### *Eastern Greek*

In the third century BC, the Greeks, led by Alexander the Great, conquered the eastern Mediterranean and as far east as India. Over the next few centuries, knowledge also spread out from Greece in all directions, and the Romans absorbed a lot of ideas from Greek culture. Greek words started to be used in Latin. There was a need to be able to write down these words.

The Romans translated most of the letters, making do with such combinations as *PH* instead of *f* and *TH* instead of *t*. But they had no way of writing two particular Greek sounds, so in about AD 100;

the Romans borrowed two letters from the Eastern Greek alphabet. One was *Υ*, which was very much the same as the *V* they had already gotten from Western Greek. In Eastern Greek it had retained a long stem, while in Western Greek it had lost it. The Eastern Greek pronunciation was by now slightly different as well, using the slender *u* sound we get in the German word *fünf* or the French *tu*. The other letter the Romans borrowed was the Zeta *Ζ*, for the *z* sound. Both the *Υ* and the *Ζ* were only used for writing Greek words, so the letters were placed at the end of the alphabet, although *Ζ* had centuries before been positioned after *F*.

So, by the time the Roman Empire reached its peak in the fourth and fifth centuries, the alphabet looked like this:

A B C D E F G H I K L M N O P Q R S T V X Y Z

Due to the Roman dominance of Europe, the Roman alphabet became the standard alphabet throughout Western Europe, and eventually it spread throughout the Western world.

## More New Letters

After the Norman invasion of Britain in the eleventh century, the Anglo-Saxon language was written down using Roman letters. There was no letter for the *w* sound in Anglo-Saxon, which didn't exist in Latin. At first, they used the runic wen, which looks like a narrow triangular *P*, but it was too easy to mix up with an actual *P*, so they started to write it using a double *U*, hence the name "double u." At that time, there was only one letter for both the vowel sound *u* and consonant sound *v*, and it looked like a *V*, so *W* looks like two *V*s. The *W* was placed in the alphabet beside the *V* to which it was related.

Another letter was introduced into English at that time, from the runic alphabet: Thorn Þ. This was used to represent the *th* sound in English. Thorn died out later on, although it is still used in Iceland. The only place you'll see it now in English is in a corrupted form as a *Υ* at the start of "Ye Olde Tea Shoppe."

The letter *U* started off as a written variation of the letter *V*. The *V* symbol represented mainly the *u* sound, but it could also be used for the *v* sound. In some forms of handwriting, *V* was written with a rounded bottom, but it still represented both the vowel *U* and the consonant *V*. Later, people started using the pointed *V* when they meant the consonant and the rounded *U* when they meant the vowel. Because these were considered to be variations of the same letter, they were put side by side in the alphabet.

The last letter to be added to the English alphabet was the letter *J*. Similarly to the evolution of *U* and *V*, *I* and *J* started out as variations of a single letter. Scribes might put a long tail on a final *I* if there were a few in a row. For example, Henry the Eighth could be written "Henry VIII" It was up to the scribe to decide which version of the letter he wanted to use.

In Rome, *I* represented both the vowel *I* and the consonantal *y* sound at the start of the English word *yellow*. Gradually over the centuries, the consonant was changed: in Spain it became an *H*, in Germany it remained a *Y*, and in France it became a *j* sound. When the Normans invaded England in 1066, they brought the *j* sound with them but continued to spell it with the letter *I*, which could be written *I* or *J* depending on which looked good.

In about the fifteenth century (around the time of the printing press), people started to fix on *I* for the vowel and the *J* for the consonant, but this was not fully accepted until the mid-seventeenth century.

So from the seventeenth century onward, our alphabet contained the same twenty-six letters as we now use. But even then, many scholars still treated it as having only twenty-four: they still considered *U* and *V* as one letter, and *I* and *J* as one letter. For example, Samuel Johnson's dictionary, published in the mid-eighteenth century, had all the *I* and *J* words mixed together. It was only in the mid-nineteenth century that scholars fully accepted that these were separate letters and that there are twenty-six letters in the alphabet. (70)

## *Conclusion of the Modern Alphabet*

With the invention of *J* (thank goodness for the *J*—my name is John, and my oldest son's name is Jay), the English alphabet contained the twenty-six letters that we know so well. Other languages in Europe added accents to many letters to cue extra sounds—for example á, Å, and Ä—but English has avoided this. There have also been attempts to revise the alphabet and introduce new letters to represent the *ng* sound, the *ee* sound, and so on. All such attempts have so far been doomed to failure. The vowels of *A-E-I-O-U* were accepted for pronunciation.

Fortunately, the alphabet reached a level of maturity just before the invention of the printing press, or readers of much of what was printed would have needed an interpreter. Likewise, the combination of printing books in a common alphabet and each country's' own language allowed each country to maintain records in its common language, not exclusively in either Greek or Roman. In this manner, education within a country could be accelerated and, with the common alphabet, could be translated into the language of other countries to further enhance the transfer of knowledge from one country to another.

The common alphabet and the printing press accelerated the spread of knowledge. The spread of knowledge beyond the sixteenth century was gigantic. To make an even bigger expansion of the world's knowledge, the New World was colonized by the leaders of the world at that time, and they brought their languages and books and teachings to the New World early in the seventeenth century.

You can appreciate the impact of the alphabet and the printing press, as they allowed solutions to problems to be documented and shared, avoiding the need to resolve the same issues time after time. I might comment that progress through the centuries has been led by the invention of some better means of communication. Examples are the phonograph, telephone, telegraph, radio, television, computer, cellular phone, FAX machine, home printer, Internet, specialty items like the iPod, iPad, and iPhone ... and the list goes on and will continue in the near future.

But other types of inventions were needed to carry man further. He needed new tools to allow him to continue his progress toward learning more about the enemies he could not see. Man was rewarded by the skills of a janitor in the country of Holland (the Netherlands) when he polished the round glasses that were to make the next giant step toward solving many of man's problems.

## The Microscope—He Polished His Lens to Make a Better Microscope.

In the next sections of this book I will discuss various additional illnesses and diseases and how they affected the world. I consider this a part of the evolution of man on earth. In a sort of backhanded way the diseases I will be discussing also spread the learning of man. Each disease that affected humans the world over resulted in communication the world over. Cures for diseases began to spread to countries other than the ones where the cures originated through books and articles. Advancements in the instruments that helped to find and cure diseases reached the peoples of the world. It seems that nothing is communicated faster than a disease that strikes or a cure that is found.

When I was in the navy, I spent the last three years off-ship stationed at the Patuxent Naval Air Station; while there, in 1954 I read a very interesting book called *Microbe Hunters*, by Paul de Kruf. (27) This book was originally published in 1926 and was republished in 1954. This thoroughly interesting book is about the invention of the microscope and how doctors and scientists used this piece of equipment from the middle of the seventeenth century through early in the twentieth century. I cover several of the scientists that were included in the book. Although I had a degree in electrical engineering and was responsible for manufacturing the first integrated circuit on silicon, and spent my life providing advances in integrated technology, there were several occurrences that got me interested in medicine and medical advances, and brought me to writing books about my experiences. In 1965 I took on a position with a new company in Massachusetts as the general manager for integrated circuits. After my physical I got a phone call from Mr. Sprague, the owner of the company. He was concerned about my blood pressure readings, and since he was on the board of Massachusetts General Hospital, he had made an appointment for me to go there that Thursday.

After a week the doctors of Mass General told me that I was not going to live long, because my blood pressure (I was thirty-three years old) was 240 over 200. They said the bottom and top readings were tearing away at my cells. Needless to say, the following year was spent each Saturday going to Mass General and trying different medicines. Most made it impossible to drive home, or I was dizzy while at work. The problem was that no matter what they gave me to take the top reading down, the bottom reading remained constant. Since the pulse pressure is directly determined by the difference between those two readings, and the bottom one didn't move while the top reading was reduced, this resulted in a reduced pulse and made me weak; sometimes to the point of passing out. After six months they found several medicines that brought my readings to 150 over 100.

In 1968 I moved to California, and my blood pressure dropped to 140 over 100 for no reason that I knew of. In 1976 I was picked up by a different doctor. He couldn't believe how I could function with those medicines in me, and he changed them. My blood pressure dropped to 125 over 80, and I have been taking that same medicine since then.

Meanwhile, I kept reading about medical advances and eventually was operated on for my gall bladder. Then in 1980 I lost my sense of taste, and the neurologist kept taking MRIs of my brain every six months to see if he could determine the reason. One visit he told me he was going to have them do an ultrasound on my neck, because he didn't like what he heard. Two days later he said my Carotid artery was 85 percent blocked and told me I should have it operated on. I asked him, "How about today?" He made some calls, and the following Monday they did an arteriogram, and on Tuesday they operated on me. Nothing seem to change medical wise.

Each of these conditions I went through brought me to studying what causes what. Each day after every meal I would wash my mouth with Listerine for thirty-five seconds, spit it out, and gargle with a mouthful of water that was diluted by the Listerine—six times. After seventeen years of no taste, I started to get my taste back and went to the doctor and asked if he knew why. He said, "It's possible that there previously was no connection between your brain and taste buds and eventually stem cells developed a new path that connected and allowed you to taste." I said, "I have been reading about stem cells, and this sounds like a possible reason." Actually, I believed that he didn't know and came up with that thought. So, as the years progressed I continued reading about medical issues; I've been reading about medical issues since 1965. It got to the point where various people would ask me if I knew something about their particular medical problems, and it turns out I was helpful to many people. I will be eighty-four in several months, and my blood pressure and cholesterol and my activities have remained in check. So I write about these things that I have learned through experience, reading, and using my computer.

The next significant achievement, one that generated a big surge in the scientific world, was the invention of the microscope. It began with the crazy love for the grinding of lenses by a Dutch janitor, Antony van Leeuwenhoek, who was born in 1632 in Delft, Holland. (27) He left school at the age of sixteen and became an apprentice in a dry goods store in Amsterdam. At the age of twenty, he left this job and went back to his hometown, married, and set up a dry goods store of his own. He had several children. Antony became very interested in the use of a microscope while reviewing cloth in his store. He used a 10x microscope, (really nothing more than a magnifying glass) which is all the world had at the time, to count the threads. He began to grind and polish his own lenses (named after the lentil because of the shape) and looked at things under his superior microscope. He did more than just provide a superior lens. His microscope was a fairly complex arrangement of the lens and the means of light passing properly through the lens. He did this for years while serving as a janitor for the town's city hall. By the age of forty he had about one hundred microscopes. When he found a way to improve one, he would return to the early versions and make changes. His interest in the various aspects of the device, such as the metals used to hold the lenses and other parts of the microscope, were evident in his lenses and scopes.

He would study a frog's leg and try to understand how every little thing worked. He observed the eyes of flies and would tell people about them. Many thought he was not of sound mind. He heated glass tubes and shaped them into needle-sized tips that allowed him to pick up very small objects.

When he was around forty years old, he went out into his yard and took a drop of water from one of his plants. He brought it into his workshop and looked at the water under his microscope. What Leeuwenhoek saw would result in the war on bacteria (although he didn't know it at the time—it would be many years before what he saw were called bacteria). He couldn't believe his eyes. There were little animals running around in the water. He wondered where they came from. He took a saucer from the cabinet and washed it and cleaned it with some chemical and looked to see if anything was on the saucer. It was clean. He then set it out in the rain and brought it in and looked and saw nothing. He took a pepper seed and placed it in the water and saw nothing. He left it to sit for a couple of days, and when he looked he saw the normal ones that he previously had seen and one very big one that seemed to be eating the smaller ones. He decided to try to find out where they came from. He would look at his saliva and be very excited to see that these little creatures were there also. One day after drinking a very hot cup of coffee, he looked at a drop of saliva and found none. He picked around in his mouth and finally found a place in a back tooth that had many. He then did experiments with hot coffee and found that it could kill the creatures; when the coffee cooled down, they remained motionless.

At about this time in history, a group of men founded a little group called The Invisible College, which would secretly meet in England to discuss things they had done or seen. These meetings had to be secret because if the men of Cromwell heard about anything like this, they would think that it was a conspiracy against the government. This group of men included Isaac Newton and Robert Boyle, who was the founder of the science of chemistry, so they were scientists of note. They began to get word that a Dutch janitor had made microscopes that allowed one to see very small creatures. They found it hard to believe and determined that this janitor had microscopes that magnified by a factor of 200, when normal ones magnified by 10. (I would like to make a note here for the reader's benefit. A microscope can only resolve things that are bigger than one-half a wavelength of light. The average wavelength of light is 0.55 micrometers. So the best microscopes that worked off of light could resolve things as small as 0.275 micrometers. If you were to look through one of Leeuwenhoek's best microscopes, which magnified by approximately 270, it would look like 75 micrometers—or three-thousandths of an inch (human hair is between three-thousandths and seven-thousandths of an inch), which is about the smallest thing that the human eye can detect. What this says to me is that his microscope in the middle of the seventeenth century was almost as good as today's microscopes.)

Newton decided to visit Leeuwenhoek. During his visit he was allowed to look through the microscopes but was not allowed to touch one. Newton was very astounded at what he saw and convinced Leeuwenhoek that he should take notes on what he found and distribute them to The Invisible College. Thus began cooperation between this janitor and the highest of high scientists of England. Leeuwenhoek would investigate many things in his life and continue until he was ninety. He died when he was ninety-one. On his deathbed, he asked his best friend to forward the last two reports that he had written. They had to be converted into Latin and sent to the Royal Society in England. The microscope of this janitor was as big an invention as the printing press, since now science could use it to visit another world of living things.

Robert Hooke, the English father of the microscope, made a copy of Leeuwenhoek's light microscope and then improved upon his design. (28) Although his microscope was easier to use than Leeuwenhoek's, he commented that his microscope didn't resolve small dimensions as well as Leeuwenhoek's. In 1678, after Leeuwenhoek had written to the Royal Society with a report of discovering "little animals"—perhaps bacteria and protozoa—Hooke was asked by the society to confirm these findings. He successfully did so, thus paving the way for wide acceptance of Leeuwenhoek's discoveries. Hooke was the author of the book *Micrographia*, which detailed the various things he had observed with very accurate drawings. His observation of the details of cork contained information that was the first description of cells. He described the cells of the cork as being like a honeycomb. Until that time there was no understanding of living things being composed of cells. Of course, without the microscope it was impossible to be aware of this. The same is true of the discovery by Leeuwenhoek of bacteria and protozoa. Hooke is credited with discovering the basic unit of life, the cell. Hooke is also credited with being the first to use the basic three-lens configuration that is still used in microscopes today. There has not been a major change in the basic light microscope in these past 330 years.

Hooke examined fossils with his microscope, the first person to do so. He noted close similarities between the structures of petrified wood and fossil shells on the one hand, and living wood and living mollusk shells on the other. Most people at the time didn't believe that fossils represented forms of life that had lived previously on earth. He described how fossils really represented previous living creatures and how they would become like these fossils. This work was done 250 years before Darwin. He described how these fossils found on high ground had previously been under water and how these remains could be used to determine the history of life.

### Improvements in the Microscope, up to the Present

I have been writing this book more or less in chronological order of things that happened and affected man's battle against disease. However, I am going to cover the improvements in the microscope regardless of time so as to bring a clearer picture to the reader.

Improvements in the resolution of microscopes required that three basic problems be resolved.

The first related to chromatic aberration, which is the unequal bending of different colors of light that occurs in a lens. (29) This was solved by Chester Hall in the 1730s by using a second lens with a different shape and light-bending properties. He found that he could realign the colors without losing the magnification of the first lens.

The second related to spherical aberration, which was solved by Joseph Jackson Lister; it relates to the unequal bending of light that hits different parts of a lens. He resolved this problem by placing the lenses at precise distances from each other, which eliminated the aberration from the first lens. Also, if a low-power, low-curvature lens could be made with minimal aberration and placed as the first lens in the series, this virtually eliminated spherical aberration.

The third problem was that for a microscope to be as good as physically possible, it must collect a cone of light that is as wide as possible. This problem was solved by Ernst Abbe with the use of water and oil immersion lenses. The maximum resolution that Abbe was able to achieve is about ten times better than the resolution that Leeuwenhoek had achieved a hundred years earlier. This resolution of 200 nanometers (0.2 micrometers) is a physical limit placed by the wavelength of light. Remember I previously mentioned that a light microscope could resolve one-half of a wavelength of light and used the average wavelength of light, which is 0.550 micrometers. The actual lower limit of light that man can see is 0.400 micrometers, so Ernst Abbe was able to take the microscope down to the lower limit, which is lower than the average wavelength previously mentioned.

### The First Electron Microscope

Instead of glass being used to bend and focus light, electron microscopes use magnetic coils to do the same thing with electrons. (29) H. Busch was the first to use a magnetic coil like a lens, in 1926. E. Ruska made the first image-producing electron microscope in 1933, which passed the 200-nanometer optical limit. Ruska and his company, Siemens of Germany, produced the first commercial electron microscope in 1939, and structures never seen before in science and engineering became visible. Much of what we know about the Nano-universe, we owe to the scanning electron microscope. There were many improvements in the electron microscope over the years. I remember in 1964 seeing Westinghouse display their improved version at the integrated circuit plant where I ran the Custom Products Group, and I could practically see inside of silicon. I was to purchase several electron microscopes over the years during the development of integrated circuits. They were much smaller in physical size, yet resolved as well as the large older ones. They also became affordable for use in industry, and their use spread rapidly.

## The First Scanning Probe Microscope

This system did not use electron beams to image a sample. Instead, it used a tiny needlelike probe that scanned back and forth across a sample's surface. The interactions were recorded into a computer to form an image. This was invented by IBM in Switzerland by Gerd Binnig and Heinrich Rohrer. They were awarded the Nobel Prize in physics in 1986 for their work. The major advantage is that this can be used without a vacuum and even in a liquid. This made three-dimensional images available with very high resolution. I had one of my groups at Micrel Semiconductor purchase one in 1993 for use in resolving very small dimensions in the development of advanced integrated circuits.

# Microscopes and the Men Who Used Them to Conquer Diseases

I covered the main advances in microscopes to the present, since they have brought medicine, biology, physics, and other sciences to the forefront over the last 365 years. With these revolutionary pieces of equipment, much could be learned about the makeup of man and how to resolve many of the diseases that could have shortened man's life on earth. I will now continue my discussion of the various advances made with the standard microscope that brought advances in life for man and discuss how the various microbe hunters battled the ailments of man.

### Spallanzani—Middle of the Eighteenth Century

Lazzaro Spallanzani was born in 1729 in a small Italian village, just six years after Leeuwenhoek died. (27) He had been educated as a scientist at the University of Reggio. He had heard of the Dutchman and began to observe the "beasties," as many called them by this time. In the mid-1700s, many scientists and others felt that the beasties came about by spontaneous generation. In other words, they felt that they were not born; they just appeared out of nowhere, spontaneously. Lazzaro didn't believe this. He did many experiments to prove this wrong. Science had advanced by this time, and there were ways to make up a soup, or culture, that would result in many beasties in a day or so. As he did his experiments, others were doing experiments to show that they could cork a flask that had the soup in it and heat it. After opening it up there were just as many beasties as before, if not more. As Spallanzani did experiments, he would take flasks and heat them and taper down the ends and then seal them off and then heat them in boiling water for different times, demonstrating that after a certain length of time, there were no beasties to be found. This would be refuted by other scientists with experiments that they conducted.

Then Spallanzani devised another experiment that he thought would prove his point. He took a tube and put beastie soup in the tube and hooked one end to a vacuum pump. Then he sealed the other end off by heating the tip again. He let it pump and pump, and no matter how much he did this, the beasties lived. He couldn't believe it. All animals had to have oxygen to live. Why were they not dead? He was befuddled.

One day Spallanzani had an idea. He went to his lab and put a cleaned glass dish under his microscope. On one side he placed a drop of the soup with the beasties and on the other side of the microscope nozzle he put a drop of clean water that had no beasties. Then he took a needle he had cleaned and stuck it in the water forming a line from the water to the clean soup. It was like making a river for the beasties to swim toward his clean water, which was under the microscope. Spallanzani then watched while the beasties moved down this line of water. When the lead beastie was under his microscope, using a very clean, fine paintbrush, he swished it through the channel of water and cut the "river" so no other beasties could swim into position under the microscope. With this deft movement he had captured one beastie under his microscope lens. He watched the beastie for hours. Then something remarkable happened. The beastie got longer and skinnier, and then there were two beasties. He continued watching; two became four, and then those four became eight. He got up and danced around his laboratory. The beasties did not appear spontaneously. Instead, each multiplied by dividing up into two beasties, and those two divided into two more, all at a rapid rate. Spallanzani had proved that the beasties were not spontaneously generated. Thus the next advance for the microbe hunters was completed.

## *Pasteur—Middle of the Nineteenth Century*

Pasteur was born in France in 1822. He attended a Paris university and received degrees in chemistry. (27) Pasteur first found the little animals in his microscope when he was trying to understand why some of France's grape crops were not producing the wine they were famous for. He viewed the good and bad wines under the microscope and found that the bad wine had no yeast in it and the good wine had yeast in it. Many experiments later, he proved to himself that the yeasts were what turned the sugar in the mix to alcohol, and that the wines that did not have these rich yeasts were devoid of these little animals he normally could see under the microscope. He proved that these little creatures were responsible for the generation of yeasts. So the little beasties could do good things as well as bad. At the time scientists didn't know the good from the bad microorganisms. Eventually, his experiments and results saved the wine industry in France.

The belief that the little beasts were formed by spontaneous generation remained. People had forgotten about Spallanzani's experiments a hundred years before and believed that the beasties appeared by spontaneous generation. Pasteur established several experiments to prove that the beasties were actually airborne and entered his mixture of broth that grew bacteria or other things by falling into the broth. It was known that if you had a clean bowl of broth and left it out for a day or two and viewed the broth, it would be full of what today we would call bacteria—they now had a proper name for the beasties. Pasteur demonstrated that the bacteria were due to the growth of microorganisms, not spontaneous generation. He exposed a bowl of boiling broth to air via a filter that prevented air particles from passing into the broth and allowed the broth to sit around for days. No bacteria could be found in the broth. He proved that the bacteria therefore came from the air as dust or spores, or were carried by other means. As soon as he removed the air filters, bacteria appeared in a short time. Through these experiments, he proved the existence of germs and developed germ theory.

Pasteur proved there were good germs and bad germs. Observing the bacteria in milk, he determined that sour milk had bad bacteria and good milk did not. He found that in milk heated to a certain temperature, the bacteria were killed while the integrity of the milk was maintained. Below that temperature, bacteria would not only remain but would multiply. If the milk were heated too high above that optimal temperature, the milk would be ruined. This was a great step toward ridding the world of problems related to milk. This process became known as pasteurization, in honor of his work. Milk pasteurization is the process of heating to eliminate harmful bacteria in milk. This is used in every qualified supplier of milk and milk products. Heat milk at 72°C (162°F) for sixteen seconds, and the bad bacteria are gone, whereas at 63°C (145°F), the milk must be heated for not less than thirty minutes. Milk is deemed pasteurized if it tests negative for alkaline phosphatase.

Pasteur's work also provided the clues necessary for providing sterile operations that were developed by other great men at that time.

Pasteur also developed methods, through the use of good bacteria, for improving wines and the yeasts that were required for other foods.

Pasteur worked on the disease that resulted in cholera in chickens. Part of this was through good fortune. The culture that had been set aside for inducing cholera in chickens mistakenly sat around for an extended period. He then injected the cholera culture into some chickens, and they didn't develop cholera. He took some new culture and tried to induce cholera in these chickens, and it failed to make the chickens sick. He went back over his work and realized that the initial culture had probably been weakened while sitting around and therefore was not strong enough to cause cholera to appear in the chickens. However, it was strong enough for the chickens to build up immunity to the disease. He repeated the experiment and proved to his satisfaction that this was indeed true. Thus through good fortune and good observation of critical details, he found a source of immunity for chicken cholera.

Later, Pasteur was to apply this same method in developing an immunization for anthrax, which affected sheep and cattle and resulted in their death. He demonstrated his anthrax cure by taking a number of cattle and giving half of them his anthrax serum, without injecting the other half. He waited a certain number of days, and then he returned. In front of a crowd of observers, he gave each of the cattle a shot of anthrax. He left the field and told the observers to return in a given period. Upon their return, the sheep, cattle, and pigs that received no serum were dead, and those that did receive the shots were walking around like nothing had happened. This proved that a vaccine could be made as he had demonstrated on chickens and cattle.

Pasteur later developed a vaccine for rabies. At the time, there was an almost 100 percent death rate in people bitten by rabid dogs. He studied how rabies developed in a dog's body and how it finally got to its brain and killed the animal. It took fourteen days for the rabies to reach the brain and kill the dog. He then took a weakened culture and injected it into a rabbit. He waited a number of days and took some blood from the rabbit and injected it into another rabbit. He kept doing this, and each rabbit eventually died. However, after a number of rabbits died, the next rabbit did not die. Microscopic study showed that the rabies carried in the blood of the animals weakened as it was passed down. He allowed dogs with rabies to bite healthy dogs, and then he gave them these shots for fourteen days, and the dogs did not become rabid.

A youngster in the neighborhood was bitten by a rabid dog, and the father appealed to Pasteur to give the boy the treatment. Although he had never tried his cure on a human, Pasteur knew the boy would die without the vaccine, so he went through with the treatment. It was a success, and the news traveled fast and far, and Pasteur was hailed as a hero.

Not long after this, a pack of wild dogs bit nineteen children in a town in Russia. The czar of Russia, hearing about Pasteur's work, sent the children to France to be treated. Pasteur was given advanced warning and realized he would not have enough time to develop the serum. He needed fourteen days with his present approach. He hurriedly changed his routine with the rabbits, giving them more rapid treatment, and provided the serum within seven days. The nineteen children were treated, and sixteen of them survived. The czar of Russia was so pleased that he provided money to build the Pasteur Research Lab in Paris, the biggest research laboratory in the world at the time. Pasteur was considered the captain of the microbe hunters.

## Koch—Late Nineteenth Century

Robert Koch began his medical practice in small towns while traveling as a young married man; then his wife brought him a microscope for his twenty-eighth birthday. He focused on studying microbes and gave less attention to his patients. (27) His first major interest was to try to find out what anthrax looked like and discover how it killed cattle and sheep. He was rather poor, and when he needed to inoculate an animal to see the results, he couldn't afford any big animals. They didn't have much room in the house where they lived, and therefore, he picked mice for his experiments. He was probably the first person to use mice to study a disease. His practice was out in the countryside, and he couldn't obtain needles to inoculate the mice. He removed the spleens from cattle that had died of anthrax, and he studied what he saw in his microscope. The bacilli he studied were motionless and looked like sticks. He wasn't sure these were what caused anthrax, but he believed they were. He made sharp sticks out of slivers of wood and collected some of these sticklike curiosities on them and injected them into the mice. The mice would die, and he would see a large number of these sticklike curiosities in their spleens. He wanted to discover if they were the actual cause of death. So he figured a way of isolating the microbes he thought were anthrax. He placed one of his sticks in a drop of the fluid from an ox's eye and placed it on a glass slide. Then he immediately put a thicker glass slide in which he had etched a depression over the culture, so that the glass wouldn't touch the culture. The thicker glass slide also had a coating of Vaseline-like material around the outside edge as a sealant. Then he very delicately turned the slide structure upside down so the culture hung in the depression. He believed that no other bacteria could then fall on the culture, even though the two glass slides should have sealed the culture from the outside world. He placed this in a homemade incubator heated by an oil lamp (remember this was a time before electricity) to body temperature and left it there for a couple of days. Then he checked it for these "sticks" that didn't move.

After several observations, he saw them move; then he saw them stretch and thin out and become two, and before long there were thousands of them under his microscope. He placed some in a drop of oxen eye fluid and repeated the experiment. He did this eight times; each time the moving sticks grew and multiplied. He injected this culture he had developed into a mouse, and the next day the mouse was dead. When he viewed its spleen, it was full of the long nonmoving sticks. He now knew that what he had taken from the original dead animals was causing death in a mouse. He was the first person to develop deadly bacteria outside of the body of an ox. He became famous for isolating the bacteria that caused tuberculosis in 1882. He repeated his performance on isolating *Vibrio cholerae* in 1883. Koch was awarded Nobel Prize in physiology and medicine for his tuberculosis findings in 1905. He is considered the father of bacteriology.

Koch also researched why anthrax would reappear after long periods had passed without problems, sometimes many years. His studies showed that when the anthrax lay in the dead body of a victim for some length of time, it then transformed into endospores that could last a long time. These spores might wait on the ground for a hundred years until cattle or sheep would breathe them in and become ravaged by this deadly disease. He announced that every animal that died needed to be burned or buried deep in the ground where the temperature is too cold for the bacteria to be active. These became the accepted procedures.

These endospores, embedded in soil, were the cause of unexplained "spontaneous" outbreaks of anthrax. Koch published his findings in 1876 and was rewarded with a job at the Imperial Health Office in Berlin in 1880. In 1881, he urged the sterilization of surgical instruments using heat.

In Berlin, he improved the methods he used in Wollstein, including staining and purification techniques and bacterial growth media, including the Petri dish, named after its inventor, his assistant Julius Richard Petri. These devices are still used today. In 1883, Koch worked with a French research team in Alexandria, Egypt, on cholera. Koch identified the *Vibrio* bacterium that caused cholera, though he never managed to prove it in experiments. The bacterium had been previously isolated by Italian anatomist Filippo Pacini in 1854, but his work had been ignored due to the predominance of the miasma theory of disease. Koch was unaware of Pacini's work and made an independent discovery. His greater status meant that the discovery would be widely spread for the benefit of others. In 1965, however, the bacterium was formally renamed *Vibrio cholerae - Pacini 1854.*

In 1885, he became professor of hygiene at the University of Berlin and later, in 1891, director of the newly formed Institute of Infectious Diseases, a position that he resigned from in 1904. He started traveling around the world, studying diseases in South Africa, India, and Java.

Probably as important as his work on tuberculosis, for which he was awarded the Nobel Prize, are Koch's postulates, which say that to establish that an organism is the cause of disease, it must be

* Found in all examined cases of the disease
* Prepared and maintained in a pure culture
* Capable of producing the original infection
* Even after several generations in culture, be retrievable from an inoculated animal and cultured again

After Koch's success, his pupils found the organisms responsible for diphtheria, typhoid, pneumonia, gonorrhea, cerebrospinal meningitis, leprosy, bubonic plague, tetanus, and syphilis, among others, using his methods.

He died on May 27, 1910, at age sixty-six. The Koch Crater on the moon was named after him. The Robert Koch Prize and Medal were created to honor microbiologists who make groundbreaking discoveries or who contribute to global health in a unique way.

The first non-German to be awarded the medal was Professor Bill Hutchison of Glasgow.

## Metchnikoff and the Phagocytes—Early Twentieth Century

Metchnikoff was born in Russia in 1845 and died in July 1916. He was accepted at Kharkov University in 1863 to study natural sciences and completed the four-year course in two years. (30)

After reading about Pasteur, he became interested in studying microbes. He began to look at starfish that he kept in his laboratory. Starfish larvae have crystal-clear bodies, and you can see what goes on inside them. Metchnikoff was watching one under a microscope when he saw something swarming through the fish's body and consuming various things. He thought that maybe the body of the fish had a built-in immune system that included these cells that gobbled up any invading microbes. He thought about the fact that after a thorn pierced a finger, the finger would soon swell with pus. He immediately made the conclusion that the pus was caused by these cells in one's body trying to rid the body of the invaders. He wondered how that would affect the starfish. He went into his garden and got a stem from a rosebush. He stuck one of the thorns in the starfish and then watched the actions of these moving creatures inside the fish. Sure enough, they swam toward the thorn and began to swallow up the intruders. He and a friend decided they had to give a name to these cells that did this work. He wanted to give them a Greek name, since Greek names are prevalent throughout science. After a time they decided on *phagocytes*, from the Greek work for "devouring cell."

Next, Metchnikoff studied water fleas, since they also have a crystal-clear body. Study showed that they also had a built-in mechanism that worked like that in the larva of the starfish.

Eventually, Metchnikoff went to the Pasteur Institute to work under the man himself. Pasteur gave him a laboratory of his own. Pasteur believed he was on the right trail toward understanding why humans didn't always die from an infection. Metchnikoff preached about phagocytes for twenty years at the research laboratory and converted many to this way of thinking. The only argument that his opposition ever gave him was that the phagocytes devoured everything, including food. But Metchnikoff always had a good argument.

Metchnikoff was awarded the Nobel Prize for medicine in 1908 for his theory on phagocytes, which are white blood cells. It was found that they do elevate immunity levels in the human body and fight infection. Some form of them are still called phagocytes.

## Oxygen and the Breathing of Air

Before I go much further into the details of the brilliant advances made by the people of science and medicine, I would like to bring to the reader's attention something that really shocked me as I reviewed these accomplishments, and this relates to oxygen.

Oxygen was discovered by Joseph Priestley and Carl Wilhelm Scheele in 1774. On August 1, 1774, Priestly focused sunlight on mercuric oxide inside a glass tube, which liberated a gas he named dephlogisticated air. (31) He noted that candles burned brighter in the gas and that a mouse was more active and lived longer while breathing it. Unknown to Priestley, Swedish pharmacist Carl Wilhelm Scheele had already produced oxygen by heating mercuric oxide and various nitrates sometime in 1772. Noted French chemist Antoine Lavoisier later claimed to have independently discovered the new substance.

My point is this: the importance of oxygen to human life was not discovered until late in the nineteenth century. The bigger shock is that it was not known that the important part of the air that humans breathe is oxygen. This was discovered just before the Civil War in the United States around 1865. My shock related to my ignorance that this was discovered so late in the life of man. I assumed we knew this. It wasn't till after the Civil War that the percentage of oxygen we breathed in and how much we breathed out was realized. Isn't that a shock when you consider all the progress made by scientists and medical doctors up to this time, who didn't know what kept us alive?

This goes to show you that one cannot take anything for granted. At times you may think you are ignorant, or dumb, or behind the times, or whatever, but don't take it that way. There is much to learn as we go through this wonder of life.

## No Lightbulbs or Lights—Beginning of the Twentieth Century

I always have to keep reminding myself that certain things were not available to man as he proceeded on his advancements. Remember there were no lightbulbs during these early times. There were candles and oil lamps. Microscopes had no lighting. Electricity was just making a big impact on the world early in the 1800s. Electric lights really started in 1900 and were not yet widespread across the country or the world. There was no central heating or air conditioning in the world, and these developments didn't make any inroads in the United States until after World War II. As you read about these accomplishments on diseases and other facets of life's improvements, keep these things in mind. Amazing accomplishments were achieved under very difficult conditions. The evolution of disease-fighting methods really became improved with the evolution of scientific methods to aid the fight against diseases. Most of these scientific methods became available as the twentieth century evolved.

# Other Microbe Hunters

There were several other microbe hunters during the last part of the nineteenth century and early twentieth century that paved the way for understanding and curing diseases. These pioneers paved the way for improving human life through their findings.

Emilee Roux (under Pasteur) and Emil von Behring (under Koch) studied the causes and cures of diphtheria (which killed 50 percent of the children struck by this disease), typhoid, pneumonia, and meningitis. They followed the procedures established by Louis Pasteur and Robert Koch (here is knowledge being passed along to ensure continuity without the necessity to learn lessons over again) with the high degree of patience required to follow every clue and every detail. Sometimes serendipity helped them identify the microbe causing the issues and develop an antitoxin that would cure disease. Their accomplishments helped to reduce the fear and destruction that prevailed where these diseases had previously run rampant.

Theobald Smith became the first American microbe hunter. (32) He was a pioneering epidemiologist and pathologist and is widely considered to be America's first internationally significant medical research scientist. He became famous for finding the cause of tick fever, or Texas fever, a debilitating cattle disease. This was an unusual disease. Cattle could be shipped to Texas from the north without problems; however, cattle that were shipped from Texas to the north came down with this disease. Smith, in 1889, discovered the tick-borne protozoan parasite responsible for Texas fever. It turned out that the cattle that were born and raised in the north were immune to tick fever, but the cattle that were transferred to the north were not immune. The adult tick would take blood from infected cattle and then drop to the ground and lay eggs. The small ticks would crawl up the legs of the cattle and transfer this disease to the cattle when feeding on blood. This was the first time that an arthropod had been definitively linked with the transmission of an infectious disease, which presaged the eventual discovery of insects as important vectors in a number of diseases.

David Bruce was a British bacteriologist born in Melbourne, Australia, in 1855. In 1894 he went to South Africa. (27) (33) For many years he searched for a cause for sleeping sickness; in 1894 he discovered the microorganism not only for that disease but also of the tsetse fly disease, as well as the method of transmission. In 1903, he went to Uganda to investigate sleeping sickness. In 1904, he proceeded to Malta to conduct additional investigations into Malta fever. In every case a great advance in the study of tropical medicine was the result. Once you find the culprit, you then can find a way to reduce its effects.

Ronald Ross, of Scottish descent, was born in India and completed his study of medicine at St. Bartholomew's Hospital in London in 1875. (27) (34) He studied malaria between 1881 and 1899. He worked on malaria in Calcutta at the Presidency General Hospital. In 1897 Ross was posted in Ootacamund and fell ill with malaria. After this he was transferred to Secunderabad, where he discovered the presence of the malarial parasite within a specific genus of mosquito, the *Anopheles*. He initially called them dapple-wings, and he was able to find the malaria parasite in a mosquito that he allowed to feed on a malaria patient named Hussain Khan. Later, using birds that were sick with malaria, he was able to ascertain the entire life cycle of the malarial parasite, including its presence in the mosquito's salivary glands. He demonstrated that malaria is transmitted from infected birds to healthy ones by the bite of the mosquito, a finding that suggested the disease's mode of transmission to humans. In 1902, Ross was awarded the Nobel Prize in physiology or medicine for his remarkable work on malaria.

## Dr. Walter Reed

Although many researchers had been trying to solve the mystery of the yellow fever epidemic throughout the nineteenth century, it was the brief Spanish-American War of 1898 that provided the pressure that resulted in a solution. [27] [35] The United States had gone to war with Spain to support rebels in Cuba and Puerto Rico who wanted to be free from violent and repressive Spanish control. The American public was particularly supportive of the rebels because of the "yellow journalism" of William Randolph Hearst, who published a series of exaggerated stories on Spanish atrocities. When the USS *Maine* was sunk in a Havana port, battle cries of "Remember the Maine" sent the United States into war against Spain. The United States defeated Spain in less than one year, because of its naval superiority. Early in the war, a severe yellow fever epidemic broke out among Cuban peasants and American soldiers stationed in Havana

For many years, scientists had struggled with solving the problem of the puzzling epidemic, but it wasn't until the outbreak of yellow fever in Havana that the problem was solved by an American-led team of scientists. The US Army was incredibly motivated by the war to halt this deadly epidemic, which could be fatal to soldiers. In an effort to find ways to control yellow fever epidemics, the US surgeon general commissioned a team of researchers, led by army medical scientist Dr. Walter Reed, to go to Cuba and accelerate all efforts to figure out how the disease spread. Dr. Reed had considered many ideas and began testing them, including looking into insects. Epidemics seemed to follow the course of wind currents, and they would stop when cold stopped mosquitoes from breeding. Dr. Reed's bold experiments proved that yellow fever was indeed spread by the bite of the mosquito *Aedes aegypti*. He had one set of volunteers sleep on the soiled clothes and beds of yellow fever patients in a room screened so that no mosquitoes could get in. None of these people contracted the disease. He had another control group of volunteers stay completely away from sick patients, except he let mosquitoes that had been allowed to feast first on people sick with the disease to bite the volunteers. These volunteers did get sick. There was no doubt; although yellow fever was not directly contagious from one person to another, it was spread by insect bites that carried it from one to another.

Dr. Reed's discovery had an immediate and powerful effect and has since rid much of the world of this horrible disease. As a result of his discovery, yellow fever patients were kept in a room with mosquito screens, and any nearby breeding grounds of the insect were destroyed. Within three months yellow fever was eliminated from Havana, for the first time in over 150 years. The same techniques were used a few years later in Panama, which had suffered epidemics. Panama has not seen even a single case since. It is widely held that it was only then possible to build the Panama Canal. This is another example of how the pressures of war can lead to a powerful and useful medical innovation.

## Paul Ehrlich, 1854–1915

Although he lacked formal training in experimental chemistry and applied bacteriology, Paul Ehrlich was introduced by his mother's cousin, the pathologist Carl Wiegert, to the technique of staining cells with chemical dyes, a procedure used to view cells under the microscope. (27) (36) While working on his medical degree, he continued to experiment with cellular staining. The selective action of these dyes on different types of cells suggested to Ehrlich that chemical reactions formed the basis of cellular processes. From this idea he reasoned that chemical agents could be used to heat diseased cells or to destroy infectious agents, a theory that revolutionized medical diagnostics and therapeutics.

After receiving his medical degree from the University of Leipzig in 1878, Ehrlich was offered a position as head physician at the prestigious Charite Hospital in Berlin. There he developed a new staining technique to identify the tuberculosis bacillus (a bacterium) that had been discovered by Robert Koch. Ehrlich also differentiated the numerous types of blood cells of the body and thereby laid the foundation for the field of hematology.

Ehrlich was a brilliant man. He read that there were only two compounds of arsenic that could be given to a rabbit without killing the rabbit. He didn't believe this and within days had already proved ten compounds of arsenic that wouldn't kill a rabbit. Between 1892 and 1910, he continued this work. He developed the best book on arsenic and arsenic compounds, which is considered the bible of arsenic. In about 1896 he claimed that one day he would find one of these compounds that wouldn't kill a rabbit but would cure syphilis. This drove him to continue his search for the "magic bullet." In 1910, he gave a rabbit that had a cancerous cell compound 606, and the rabbit not only survived but got better within days. Ehrlich had his magic bullet: number 606 of the compounds of arsenic.

Here not only was a disease that was a killer, but men and women who got syphilis were also cast out and thought of as dirty. This disease was worldwide and was spread by the love of man rather than the hate of man. A person that had this disease would only require one shot of the arsenic compound to be better by the next day. No medicine had ever had such an immediate impact as this. It was called Salvarsan. Ehrlich's biggest problem was having enough of the medicine produced. He had to teach the pharmaceutical companies that began supplying the medicine to doctors the world over. This medicine proved effective for many years.

### Joseph Lister, 1827–1912

Lister attended the University of London. In 1854, Lister became first assistant surgeon to James Syme at the University of Edinburgh in Scotland. After six years he got a professorship of surgery at the University of Glasgow. (37)

Hospital wards were occasionally aired out at midday, but Florence Nightingale's doctrine of fresh air was seen as science fiction. Facilities for washing hands or the patients' wounds did not exist, and it was even considered unnecessary for the surgeon to wash his hands before he saw a patient.

Lister became aware of a paper published by Louis Pasteur that demonstrated that rotting and fermentation could occur without any oxygen if microorganisms were present. Lister confirmed this with his own experiments. If microorganisms were causing gangrene, the problem was how to get rid of them. Pasteur suggested three methods: to filter them out, to heat them up, or to expose them to chemical solutions. The first two were inappropriate in a human wound, so Lister experimented with the third.

Carbolic acid (phenol) had been in use as a means of deodorizing sewage, so Lister tested the results from spraying instruments, surgical incisions, and dressings with a solution of it. Lister found that carbolic acid solution swabbed on wounds markedly reduced the incidence of gangrene, and he subsequently published a series of articles. "Antiseptic Principle of the Practice of Surgery" described this procedure in the journal *The Lancet* on March 16, 1867.

He also made surgeons wear clean gloves and wash their hands with 5 percent carbolic acid solutions before and after operations. Also, he first persuaded Charles Goodyear to manufacture rubber gloves for his nurse, since the carbolic acid caused her to suffer from contact dermatitis. Instruments were also washed in the same solution, and assistants sprayed the solution in the operating theater. One of his recommendations was to stop using porous natural materials in the manufacture of the handles of medical instruments.

As the germ theory of disease became more widely accepted, it was realized that infection could be better avoided by preventing bacteria from getting into wounds in the first place. This led to the rise of sterile surgery. Some consider Lister "the father of modern antisepsis." Listerine mouthwash is named after him for his work in antisepsis.

Lister moved from Scotland to King's College Hospital in London and became the second man in England to operate on a brain tumor. He also developed a method of repairing kneecaps with metal wire and improved the technique of mastectomy. His discoveries were greatly praised, and he was made Baron Lister of Lyme Regis and became one of the twelve original members of the Order of Merit.

## Other Major Impacts of the Nineteenth Century

I cannot leave the nineteenth century without covering three major contributions made by three men during that century. These three contributed significantly to the progress of man and did so without specifically working on diseases or illness, though their work did indirectly affect these areas. The three that made contributions with their work were Gregor Mendel, on the basics of genetics; Charles Darwin, on the theory of evolution; and Oliver Wendell Holmes, on hygiene.

## Gregor Mendel and Genetics

The scientist known as the father of genetics is Gregor Mendel. (38) Born in July of 1822 in what is known today as the Czech Republic, Mendel pursued various studies of science from 1851 to 1853; however, he converted and became a monk at the age of twenty-one. Remember when I was discussing religion and mentioned that there were those who spent their lives dedicated to working on other things besides religion. These were the monks in the monasteries. Here was one of the most famous, although it wasn't recognized for years after he was dead.

Gregor Mendel played a very important role in the discovery of genes and heredity. He is considered to be the father of genetics, known for his famous experiments on peas that explained the patterns of inheritance.

He began his famous hybrid cultivation of pea plants in the year 1856. Mendel originally hypothesized that in every generation, a plant inherits two "units of information" (they were not called genes at the time) for a trait, one from each parent. He carried out his experimental work in the monastery garden. At first the cultivation resulted in unpredictable results, but after careful work, Mendel noticed certain similarities when breeding the plants, such as patterns among plant generations involving dependent factors such as stem length, stalk height, round or wrinkled seeds, and other characteristics. He cross-fertilized two true-breeding pea plants, one with purple flowers and one with white flowers, and observed the offspring's characteristics; both had purple flowers. Then he let the offspring self-fertilize, and he saw that some flowers were white, but purple predominated. He continued to let the pea plants self-fertilize. Eventually he saw that his hypothesis was correct. Both "units of information" from each parent flower existed, and one trait was dominant—in this case the purple one. After spending eight years working on various plants, including upwards of twenty-eight thousand different experiments of this nature, he wrote a set of rules, or primary tenets, relating to the transmission of hereditary characteristics from parent organisms to their children. It underlies much of what is known as genetics today.

Mendel's experiments resulted in his making rules for the field of study based on his work. Mendel reasoned an organism for genetic experiments should have the following:

* A number of different traits that can be studied
* A plant should be self-fertilizing and have a flower structure that limits accidental contact
* Offspring of self-fertilized plants would be fully fertile

Mendel's experimental organism was a common pea, which has a flower that lends itself to self-pollination. The male parts of the flower are called the anthers. They produce pollen, which contains the male gametes (sperm). The female parts of the flower are the stigma, style, and ovary. The egg (female gamete) is produced in the ovary. The process of pollination (the transfer of pollen from anther to stigma) occurs prior to the opening of the pea flower. The pollen grain grows a pollen tube, which allows the sperm to travel through the stigma and style, eventually reaching the ovary. The ripened ovary wall becomes the fruit (the pea pod). Since pea plants are self-pollinators, the genetics of the parent can be more easily understood. Mendel tested all thirty-four varieties of peas available to him through seed dealers. As was previously indicated, these studies took eight years.

In February 1865, he presented his findings to the Natural History Society of Brunn, calling them "Experiments in Plant

Hybridization." No one seemed interested in Mendel's findings. He tried again, sending his work to Professor Karl von Nageli at the University of Munich, but success did not come. Mendel's results were largely neglected: though they were not completely unknown to biologists of the time, they were not seen as important. Even Mendel himself did not see their ultimate applicability and thought they only applied to certain categories of species. Despite his accomplishments, his labor would not be appreciated and recognized until thirty-four years later, when his work was rediscovered by several scientists in Europe. It was recognized that he did not merely study hybridization, but also worked with the heredity of the plants. He had developed the "rule of three," whereby the third-generation offspring would result in the dominant characteristic reappearing. I would like to interject here that I am a perfect example of this phenomenon. I am a twin, and my parents had two sets of twin boys. Three generations later, my son and his wife had a set of twin boys. This is three generations from my parents.

When Mendelian inheritance tenets were integrated with the chromosome theory of inheritance by Thomas Hunt Morgan in 1915, they became the core of classical genetics. Mendel's experiments brought forth two generalizations, which later became known as Mendel's Laws of Heredity, or Mendelian inheritance. These are described in his essay "Experiments on Plant Hybridization," which was read to the Society of Brno on February 8 and March 8, 1865, and was published in 1866. (71)

The "rediscovery" made Mendelism an important but controversial theory. Its most important promoter in Europe was William Bateson, who coined the terms *genetics*, *gene* (containing information), and *allele* (gene types) to describe many of its tenets. The model of heredity was highly contested by other biologists because it implied that heredity was discontinuous, in opposition to the apparently continuous observable variations. Many biologists also dismissed the theory because they were not sure it would apply to all species, and there seemed to be very few true Mendelian characters in nature. However, later work by biologists and statisticians such as R. A. Fisher showed that if multiple Mendelian factors were involved for individual traits, they could produce diverse amounts of results observed in nature. Thomas Hunt Morgan and his assistants would later integrate the theoretical model of Mendel with the chromosome theory of inheritance, in which the chromosomes of cells were thought to hold the actual hereditary particles, and create what is now known as classical genetics, which was extremely successful and cemented Mendel's place in history.

Mendel's findings allowed other scientists to simplify the emergence of traits to mathematical probability. A large portion of Mendel's findings can be traced to his choice to start his experiments only with true-breeding plants. He also only measured absolute characteristics such as color, shape, and position of the offspring.

His data were expressed numerically and subjected to foresight to examine several successive generations of his pea plants and record their variations. Without his careful attention to procedure and detail, Mendel's work could not have had the impact it made on the world of genetics.

The law of segregation, also known as Mendel's first law, essentially has four parts. (72)

Alternative versions of genes account for variations in inherited characteristics. This is the concept of alleles. Alleles are different versions of genes that impart the same characteristic. For example, each human has a gene that controls eye color, but there are variations among these genes in accordance with the specific color for which the gene "codes."

For each characteristic, an organism inherits two alleles, one from each parent. This means that when somatic cells are produced from two alleles, one allele comes from the mother and one from the father. These alleles may be the same (true-breeding organisms) or different (hybrids). (73)

If the two alleles differ, then one, the allele that encodes the dominant trait, is fully expressed in the organism's appearance; the other, the allele encoding the recessive trait, has no noticeable effect on the organism's appearance. In other words, only the dominant trait is seen in the phenotype of the organism. This allows recessive traits to be passed on to offspring even if they are not expressed. Not all traits have a dominant-recessive relationship, however. There is also codominance; for example, human blood types, where A and B are codominant and O is recessive.

The two alleles for each characteristic segregate during gamete production. This means each gamete will contain only one allele for each gene. This allows the maternal and paternal alleles to be combined in the offspring, ensuring variation.

The law of independent assortment, also known as "inheritance law" or Mendel's second law, states that the inheritance pattern of one trait will not affect the inheritance pattern of another. (72) While his experiments with mixing one trait always resulted in a 3:1 ratio between dominate and recessive phenotypes, Mendel's experiments with mixing two traits (dihybrid cross) showed 9:3:3:1: ratios. His 9:3:3:1 table shows that each of the two genes is independently inherited with a 3:1 ratio. Mendel concluded that different traits are inherited independently of each other, so that there is no relation, for example, between a cat's color and tail length. This is actually only true for genes that are not linked to each other.

### Rationale for These Laws

The reason for these laws is found in the nature of the cell nucleus, in our chromosomes. (I will cover human cells and chromosomes later in the book when I cover DNA; it will include discussions concerning the nucleus, where the DNA is located, and how it affects human traits.)

The cell nucleus is made up of several chromosomes carrying genetic traits. In a normal cell each chromosome has two parts, the chromatids. However, during reproduction, a reproductive cell, which is created in a process called *meiosis*, usually contains only one chromatid (half the total chromosomes of the human cell; twenty-three instead of the forty-six chromosomes in each human cell) from the chromosomes from one party and one set of chromatids from the other party. By merging two of these cell chromatids (usually one male and one female), the full set is restored and the genes are mixed. The resulting cell becomes a new embryo. The fact that this new life has half the genes of each parent is one reason for the Mendelian laws. The second, most important, reason is the varying dominance of different genes, causing some traits to appear unevenly instead of averaging out (whereby dominant doesn't mean more likely to reproduce—recessive genes can become the most common also).

There are several advantages of this method (sexual reproduction) over reproduction without genetic exchange. Instead of nearly identical copies of an organism, a broad range of offspring develops, allowing more varied abilities and evolutionary strategies.

There are usually errors in every cell nucleus. Copying the genes usually adds more of them. By distributing them randomly over different chromosomes and mixing the genes, such errors will be distributed unevenly over the various offspring. Some will therefore have very few such problems. This helps reduce problems with copying errors somewhat. This effect is supported by the chromatids of half of one sex partner mixing with the chromatids of the other partner. This rather random distribution is what helps prevent the carrying forward of errors.

Genes can spread faster from one part of a population to another. This is useful, for instance, if there's a temporary isolation of two groups. New genes developing in each of the populations don't get reduced to half when one side replaces the other; they mix and form a population with the advantages of both sides.

Sometimes a mutation (for example, sickle-cell anemia) can carry positive side effects (in this case malaria resistance). The mechanism behind the Mendelian laws can make it possible for some offspring to carry the advantages without the disadvantages, until further mutations solve the problems.

## Mendelian Trait

A Mendelian trait is one that is controlled by a single locus and shows a simple Mendelian inheritance pattern. (73) In such cases, a mutation in a single gene can cause a disease that is inherited according to Mendel's laws. Examples include sickle-cell anemia, Tay-Sachs disease, cystic fibrosis, and xeoderma pigmentose. A disease controlled by a single gene contrasts with a multifactorial disease, like arthritis, which is affected by several loci (and the environment), as well as those diseases inherited in a non-Mendelian fashion. The Mendelian Inheritance in Man database is a catalog of, among other things, genes in which Mendelian mutations cause disease.

## Charles Darwin: The Theory of Evolution

The theory of evolution, formalized by Charles Darwin, is as much a theory as is the theory of gravity, or the theory of relativity. Unlike theories of physics, biological theories—and especially evolution—have been argued long and hard in sociopolitical arenas. (39) Even today, evolution is not often taught in primary schools. However, evolution is the binding force of all biological research. It is the unifying theme. In paleontology, evolution gives scientists a powerful way to organize the remains of past life and better understand the one history of life. The history of thought about evolution in general and paleontological contributions specifically is often useful to the scientists of today. Science, like any iterative process, draws heavily from its history.

Charles Robert Darwin (1809 –82) was an English naturalist. After becoming eminent among scientists for his fieldwork and inquiries into geology, he proposed and provided scientific evidence that all species of life have evolved over time from one of a few common ancestors, through the process of natural selection.

The fact that evolution occurs became accepted by the scientific community and the general public in his lifetime, while his theory of natural selection came to be widely seen as the primary explanation of the process of evolution in the 1930s. It now forms the basis of modern evolutionary theory. In modified form, Darwin's scientific discovery remains the foundation of biology, as it provides a unifying logical explanation for the diversity of life.

Darwin's five-year voyage on the ship the *Beagle* established him as a geologist whose observations and theories supported Charles Lyell's uniformitarian ideas, and publication of his journal of the voyage made him famous as a popular author. (74) Puzzled by the geographical distribution of wildlife and fossils he collected on the voyage; Darwin investigated the transmutation of species and conceived his theory of natural selection in 1838. Having seen others attacked as heretics for such ideas, he confided only in his closest friends and continued his extensive research to meet anticipated objections. In 1858, Alfred Russel Wallace sent him an essay describing a similar theory, causing the two to publish their theories early in a joint publication.

His 1859 book *On the Origin of Species* established evolution by common descent as the dominant scientific explanation of diversification in nature. He examined human evolution and sexual selection in *The Descent of Man* and *Selection in Relation to Sex*, followed by *The Expression of the Emotions in Man and Animals*. His research on plants was published in a series of books, and in his final book he examined earthworms and their effects on soil.

Darwin's journey on the *Beagle* took him to South America and the islands around South America. During this expedition, he spent most of his time as a geologist, but from his findings he began his work on the evolution of species. (75)

The *Beagle* survey took five years, two-thirds of which was spent on land. He carefully noted a rich variety of geological features, fossils, and living organisms, and he methodically collected an enormous number of specimens, many of them new to science. At intervals during the voyage he sent specimens to Cambridge, together with letters about his findings, and these established his reputation as a naturalist. On their first stop ashore at St. Jago, Darwin found that a white band high in the volcanic rock cliffs consisted of baked coral fragments and shells. This matched Lyell's concept of land slowly rising or falling and gave Darwin a new insight into the geological history of the island that inspired him to think of writing a book on geology. [74] He went on to make many more discoveries, some of them particularly dramatic. In South America, Darwin found and excavated rare fossils of gigantic extinct mammals in strata with modern seashells, indicating recent extinction without changes in climate or signs of catastrophe. In Argentina, he found that two types of rhea had separate but overlapping territories. On the Galápagos Islands, he collected mockingbirds and noted that they were different depending on which island they came from. He also heard that local Spaniards could tell from their appearance on which island tortoises originated. (This gave him some support of what he had found, that the birds of the same species were slightly different on each of the islands. This provided him thought for the fact that the birds each had a change in their genetic structure to accommodate the weather differences on the various islands.) But he thought the creatures had been imported by buccaneers. When organizing his notes on the return journey, Darwin wrote that if his growing suspicions about the mockingbirds and tortoises were correct, "such facts undermine the stability of Species"; then he cautiously added *would* before *undermine*. He later wrote that such facts "seemed to me to throw some light on the origin of species." (74)

Captain FitzRoy was committed to writing the official narrative of the *Beagle* voyages, and near the end of the voyage, he read Darwin's diary and asked him to rewrite this journal to provide the third volume, on natural history.

### Inception of Darwin's Evolutionary Theory

In mid-December of 1859, Darwin moved to Cambridge to organize work on his collections and rewrite his journal. He wrote his first paper, showing that the South American landmass was slowly rising, and with Lyell's enthusiastic backing read it to the Geological Society of London on January 4, 1837. On the same day, he presented his mammal and bird specimens to the Zoological Society. The ornithologist John Gould soon revealed that the Galápagos birds that

Darwin had thought a mixture of blackbirds and finches were, in fact, separate species of finches. In February, Darwin was elected to the Council of the Geographical Society, and in his presidential address, Lyell presented Owen's findings on Darwin's fossils, stressing geographical continuity of species as supporting uniformitarian ideas. Gould now revealed that the Galápagos mockingbirds from different islands were separate species, not just varieties, and the wrens were yet another species of finches. Darwin had not kept track of which islands the finch specimens were from, but he found information from the notes of others on the *Beagle*, including FitzRoy, who had more carefully recorded their own collections. The zoologist Thomas Bell showed that the Galápagos tortoises were native to the islands. By mid-March, Darwin was convinced that creatures arriving in the islands had become altered in some way to form new species on the different islands, and he investigated transmutation, while noting his speculations in his "Red Notebook," which he had begun on the *Beagle*.

The question of human evolution had been taken up by his supporters (and detractors) shortly after the publication of *The Origin of Species*, (75) but Darwin's own contribution came more than ten years later with the two-volume *The Descent of Man*, and *Selection in Relation to Sex*, published in 1871. In the second volume, Darwin introduced in full his concept of sexual selection to explain the evolution of human culture; the differences between the human sexes; and the differentiation of humans, as well as the beautiful (and seemingly nonadoptive) plumage of birds. A year later Darwin published his last major work, *The Expression of the Emotions in Man and Animals*, which focused on the evolution of human psychology and its continuity with behavior of animals. He developed his ideas that the human mind and cultures were developed by natural and sexual selection, an approach that has been revived in the last three decades with the emergence of evolutionary psychology. As he concluded in *Descent of Man*, Darwin felt that, despite all of humankind's "noble qualities" and "exalted powers," "Man still bears in his bodily frame the indelible stamp of his lowly origin."

His evolution-related experiments and investigations culminated in books on the movement of climbing plants, insectivorous plants, cross-self-fertilization of plants, different forms of flowers on plants of the same species, and *The Power of Movement in Plants*. In his last book, he returned to the effects earthworms have on soil formation.

He died in Downe, Kent, England, on April 19, 1882. He had expected to be buried in St Mary's churchyard at Downe, but at the request of Darwin's colleagues, William Spotswood (president of the Royal Society) arranged for Darwin to be given a state funeral and to be buried in Westminster Abbey, close to John Herschel and Isaac Newton. (74) Darwin's works and books provided scientists with a baseline to work from, both for and against his theories. Without his work, the general subject was fairly mixed up and confusing. However, Darwin's works brought many into the subject and gave them much argumentative material to work from. However, as time went on many in the scientific community came to agree with Darwin's work. The combination of his work and the work of Mendel on genetics gave many scientists baseline work in the twentieth century to do mathematical studies of these issues. Mendel's work on peas had preceded the work of Darwin, and when scientists began to put two and two together, they could see where Mendel's work provided reasons why animals and humans could evolve with slight differences and eventually into evolution.

Many still argue against Darwin's theories, but as time passes, the evidence points toward his theory.

### The Importance of Human Hygiene

The greatest American medical genius was Dr. Oliver Wendell Holmes (1809–94) from Harvard University. (76) He was also father of the greatest American justice, Oliver Wendell Holmes. Dr. Holmes stated before he died, "Hygiene will always remain the most important discovery in medical history."

No one listened, and disease continued to rage across the United States, where the average life span was thirty-nine years. Dr. Holmes enforced hand-washing and hygiene in his son, Oliver. When Oliver Jr. was on the Supreme Court at ninety-two years, aging in splendid intellectual condition, all the other justices marveled. Justice Holmes replied, "My father taught me the vital importance of hygiene, despite my many objections at the time."

Today 99 percent of Americans have poor personal hygiene and fail to understand the consequences, although they are told, "Always wash your hands after doing anything where your hands are used or after being among large numbers of people."

It is important to understand why washing of the hands is effective in reducing various diseases. It has been found with the latest microscopes that one teaspoon of the various inhabitants on the hand contains a number or organisms greater than all the people in the world. That's a dramatic number and increases the chances that one or several on a person's hands will result in some form of medical issue. Yet when one reviews what happens when one washes his or her hands it is understood why this is effective in helping to reduce health issues. Washing the hands in soap and water results in the soap lifting the contaminants off the surface of the skin and the water rinsing it away. Doctors wash their hands and follow this by washing them some more. With each washing action more and more of the contaminants are removed. In this way the doctors enter an operation with hands with almost no foreign material that can affect the patient. This action occurring since the start of the twentieth century saw the biggest drop in infections in history.

One section of the health history of the world shines above all others: hygiene. Consider: the caveman had wonderful exercise, fresh air, no pollution, plenty of nutrients, wide diet, calorie restriction, plenty of sleep, and no modern-day stress, yet the typical life span was nineteen years. One hundred and fifty years ago, the average life span in the United States and Europe was only thirty-eight years. The average life span curve was fairly flat from 1800 to 1900, and then a big change occurred. This change in the curve is believed to be the result of several things, one of which was better hygiene. The move to better hygiene came as a result of overcoming the idea that people shouldn't wash their hands or take a bath because doing so opened the pores and allowed germs to enter the body. In England, where the idea that bathing just opened pores to let germs in prevailed, the work by various microbe hunters showed that cleaning areas of the body eliminated many of the surface germs. It is hard to imagine that the queen had a bath at birth, and bathed only two other times in her life before 1900. "Three baths in a lifetime" reflected the general public's notions that germs entered opened pores.

Results of Lister's focus on the cleanliness of surgical equipment helped to convince people, since it was proved that using Lister's approach; including cleaning all instruments and having everyone clean their hands before operating, showed a definite trend toward reduced death after operations. Hygiene began to be taught in the schools in developed countries. This included washing hands each morning, after any work, before and after a meal, and before going to bed at night. Brushing of the teeth and using mouth rinses are known to have helped not only teeth, but health in general. Practices of extra cleaning when there was a sickness in the general area helped. Another related thing that helped was the installation of drains in homes and workplaces, as well as improved sewers. These improved drains and sewers moved contamination from around the home to areas of cleanup. Proper sewage plants treated the water being carried from the homes and sent it on its way to rivers, lakes, or oceans in a proper condition.

The average life span increased as a result to around forty-nine in 1920. In the late 1970s, it reached seventy. Today the average life span in the world is seventy-nine years. Much of the improvement is the result of good hygiene. Today, in Japan the average person can expect to reach ninety in sound health, with a good mind. The magic is hygiene, and super-hygiene will help you achieve a maximum life span that may eventually exceed 125 years. It is also believed that proper diets and nutrients help us achieve longer life. A recent article in *Time* magazine discusses how the world can get to an average life span of 142 years.

Advances in sanitation, nutrition, and medical knowledge made possible improved life expectancy in the United States and throughout the world. In the United States, only 50 percent of children born in

1900 could reasonably hope to reach the age of fifty. Life expectancy improved immensely during the twentieth century, and this will be covered in the later parts of this book.

Many common sicknesses—like the common cold and ear, nose, and throat infections—would be greatly reduced if everyone washed their hands more often. The latest articles state that using soap and water is still the best method for elimination of bacteria from the body. The soap lifts the bacteria away from the skin surface, and then the water carries the soap and bacteria to the water drain. It's a fact that "germs do not fly, they hitchhike," as some wise man once said. Germs pass from one person to another when a dirty hand touches a doorknob and someone then touches that knob. The second person then carries it to the next rendezvous. Washing would have caught that germ. It's interesting that bacteria can lie around for ages in a dormant stage but then be picked up and activated many years later. Bacteria don't need to be on a live host to live. They can wait. Remember the section on anthrax? It can wait in the ground for centuries until a cow happens to eat some when feeding in the fields—and bingo, it can start right up. A virus is a different issue; it needs a host to live. It is a parasite and needs to be carried around to the next host in a short time. It is quite effective in crowds of people, since they breathe out the virus and another person can breathe it in. It cannot live long—a matter of seconds in most cases. A virus can be stopped from spreading by the practice of segregating the sick from all others for a length of time (quarantine) while the sick are being treated.

It is important to keep in mind that life expectancy averages include infant mortality in the numbers. The life expectancy figures also include women who lose their lives during childbirth. There has been considerable improvement in both of these areas. Infant mortality has been improved due to better sanitation in the hospitals and because more children are born in the hospitals instead of at home. The life expectancy for women has improved considerably, since many women use to die during childbirth. The invention of sulfa drugs almost completely eliminated the death of the woman during childbirth in the twentieth century. If the child and mother survived past the newborn's infancy, then the life expectancy for both increased dramatically. The reasons for the reduction of mothers dying during and after childbirth are covered in a later section of this book.

A good example of how things spread via the hitchhiker method is evident when a family has a couple of children in school; almost instantly the child starts having illnesses and bringing them home, and then the parents get the illness. When the kids are all through school and away at college, the health of their parents improves immensely. Young people who have no children are in better health because they don't have a child in school hitchhiking germs into their home. Much of this can be improved if the family instills good hygiene practices in their children, as well as if the children and parents wash their hands upon the child's return home. Good hygiene goes on for life. You don't grow out of needing to follow good hygiene habits. Unfortunately, underdeveloped countries don't have the facilities to meet these hygiene goals. They have no clean bathrooms, good drainage systems, chlorinated water supplies, soap, or water. The rest of the world could help the undeveloped countries by supplying them the facilities and materials to help them immediately.

# The Twentieth Century— War Starts the search for Causes and Cures of Infections

Early in the twentieth century improvements in life expectancy came from the contributions of doctors and scientists made during the nineteenth century. Illnesses such as tuberculosis, diphtheria, pneumonia, cholera, and meningitis were caused by bacteria, and with the aid of the microscope cures were developed. Cures for sicknesses caused by parasites such as the mosquito, including yellow fever, were also discovered. However, during the first thirty-one years of the twentieth century, not much additional progress was made against bacterial infections. Most of the early part of the twentieth century showed improvements due to the installation of sanitary methods in hospitals, improved hygiene in homes, and improvements in the treatment of sewage and the installation of sewage drains in homes.

However, significant progress was about to be made. As I previously mentioned, wars bring bad and good to the world. The bad is obvious, and the good can only come from the fact that much is seen by medical people during war, leading to concentrated efforts to overcome these newfound problems. This is the learning curve that it seems we must follow; that is, to make the best out of the worst. Man was now to have another chance at following this learning curve, as a war broke out in Europe. This soon became a world war, and many countries and many people were involved. As is the case with war, the medical people tried to cure and save the many wounded, which involved concentrated efforts on many levels.

During World War I, in 1914, the German army advanced to just outside of Paris, France, and the battle was fought between the two countries, with the English also helping on the side of France. Eventually the United States would enter the war. This war was a war of attrition, as the battles were fought between the trenches just north of Paris. This part of the war lasted an eternity for some, and those were the ones that were not wounded or hurt in any way. Others were not so lucky. During the three years of the battles in the trenches above Paris, eleven million soldiers died. It was a frustration of sorts, this loss of life. Most of the soldiers died not due to a direct kill by a bullet, but from the infections that followed any kind of wound. It might be nothing more than a scratch: a bullet that skimmed off a person, the nick of a bayonet on an arm or leg. In some cases, there was no visible wound to take care of, as the war in the trenches resulted in sloppy, muddy, filthy, and contaminated conditions. When a soldier was wounded in the early phases of these battles and his flesh was opened in some manner, the treatment was to pour some alcohol on the wound and sew it up. Later it was found that this was almost surely a death sentence. It was found that it was better to leave the wound alone, open, and almost unattended. It seemed the body took care of itself better in such cases. Why? That was the question.

The answer was there. The doctors and medical people on both sides of the trenches knew what was killing the soldiers; it was infection. (41) *Staphylococcus* and *Streptococcus* were the enemies, more so than the soldiers on each side of the trenches. The weather didn't help. It was damp and ideal for disease, especially these two bacteria, which seemed to be able to generate infections rapidly in the sloppy, muddy trenches. By the end of the war there were eleven million deaths, and nine million were due to infection.

### Gerhard Domagk—Learn How to Overcome These Bacterial Diseases.

One of the medical people on the German side of the trenches was Gerhard Domagk, who was witness to this terrible loss of life. He had only about a year of medical training before he was sent to the front to take care of the wounded. After what appeared to be dramatic operations on the wounded that he felt the patients would survive, in a couple of days the wounded man awakened to pain; the carefully closed incisions were now swollen, red, and painful. They gave off a foul odor, and dark liquid oozed out of the incision of the wound that he thought was healing the day before. The skin around the wound would take on a half-gelled look and puff up. This is what the physicians feared, since this was the first sign of gangrene. In this state it was called Gasbrand, for gas gangrene caused by a bacterial infection. If one of the doctors passed his gloved hand across this area, it would crackle from the rotting tissue that was releasing gas, causing the crackling. (47) This meant amputation of the limb or death. Sometimes one amputation was followed by another amputation. If nothing could stop the infection, the wounded would become silent and die of green-black gangrene.

Gas gangrene was furiously contagious, especially as it progressed. It would cause such things as leg swelling, and then came hard sores that cracked and released a gas. The gas was able to spread the bacteria to others. Once the infection was set loose in a medical ward, the patients were now isolated in wards filled with others suffering from the same fate. Going into a Gasbrand ward was like walking among the walking or lying dead. Gerhard Domagk was witness to this dreadful scene. After spending his time on the line, Gerhard was transferred to Belgium as a medical aide, joining the German troops that were readying for their offensive. Now Domagk met another silent death. Remember the flu epidemic I described in an earlier part of this book. It reached throughout the world in 1918 and lasted about eighteen months. This flu was not a part of the war, but the war spread it. Soldiers were crowded into different modes of transportation and eventually into the trenches. Soldiers were dying from the flu or from staph infections or strep infections. All of this was depressing for a medical technician. For the Germans, if the medical problems were not enough, they now were being pounded backward to whence they came, and soon the war ended.

The war ended for the soldiers, but not for Gerhard. He enrolled at Kiel University in the north of Germany to work on his medical degree. He wanted to learn how to fight the diseases he had seen in the war. In 1921, Domagk, age twenty-six, graduated from medical school. He received a *sehr gut*, the highest possible mark for his doctoral dissertation on the biochemistry of muscle cells. Gerhard worked in the laboratory of the University of Munster until 1927. He began to become discouraged because his work wasn't being recognized, even though he wrote several papers about the interactions of the body and bacteria. However, Heinrich Horlein from Bayer Chemical had read his papers. Bayer was now expanding their pharmaceutical research programs, and he contacted Gerhard. Horlein had been given the go-ahead to construct a new research building, including a state-of-the-art laboratory for pathology. Bayer had sold the Bayer aspirin brand to a US company, Sterling Products, but eventually became part of IG Farben, which was the biggest corporation in Germany. With this muscle, Bayer was in a better position to grow after the war. Gerhard Domagk was offered the position as director of experimental pathology. In 1927 he joined this company with research muscle.

Bayer was big and profitable, largely because of their dye business. They manufactured dye for almost every enterprise that required dye. Most importantly, it was the biggest supplier of dye used to stain microbes, including bacteria, and other minute things. This gave Gerhard a great starting point. He figured if the dye could stain bacteria, then he should be able to use the dye to carry various selected compounds into the cells of the body where the bacteria were doing their worst. He began the long and tedious task of finding what could attack *Staphylococcus* and *Streptococcus*.

### *Gerhard Domagk's Battle to Find a Cure for* Staphylococcus *and* Streptococcus

This war that Gerhard Domagk fought was his war in the small confines of a laboratory, staining with various compounds to identify and hopefully attack these bacteria. He was especially interested in the fact that different dyes stained different kinds of tissues. He benefited because Paul Ehrlich (the scientist previously introduced who invented the "magic bullet") was with the company, and he worked with the other scientists to develop dyes that were magic for people like Paul Ehrlich. The microscope was every bacteriologist's central instrument, but it had a terrible drawback; much of the microscopic world still could not be seen. Under a microscope, water was transparent, serum was transparent, white blood cells looked like clear blobs, and bacteria were ghosts. The solution was dye. Properly stained with some of the new synthetic dyes chemists were making from coal tar, human cells and bacteria popped out of the background, showing cell walls, nuclei, and granules preferentially. They were somehow matched. You could stain bacteria one color and the human tissue around it another. Domagk had a brilliant assistant in his war on infection.

Domagk was fortunate in that he had a great chemist working with him over the years as he tried different compounds with the various dyes. If one compound didn't work, he would feed that information back to Josef Klarer. Klarer and Domagk turned out to be a good team, with Klarer working out the chemical compounds on paper and then in actual fact. Klarer was reputed to be something of a genius; tall and a few years younger than Domagk, he was hired as part of the same 1927 expansion as was Domagk. Klarer had received his doctorate summa cum laude in Munich under the tutelage of Hans Fischer, himself a Nobel laureate. Observers had called Klarer's thesis on dye structures "sensational." He seemed destined for a stellar career in academia, but had, it was said, turned down a professorship to come to Bayer. He was brilliant but also, as brilliant people often tends to be, slightly unstable. (47)

Some chemists were theoretical, carefully thinking through structures but clumsy in the lab. Klarer, by contrast, was a natural hands-on scientist with an inborn genius for lab work—a Mozart at the bench. Many chemists worked slowly and deliberately; Klarer was spontaneous and fast. He worked without any apparent plan, and he made it look easy. Yet there was something manic about him. At Bayer he could be found toiling fiercely at all hours. He ate irregularly and disappeared for days at a time. He avoided talking with people and seemed gruff and touchy when forced into conversation. In the absence of communication, his coworkers gossiped. Klarer never slept. He had been severely wounded in the war and had undergone a long convalescence. Most of his colleagues left him alone. The tradition at Bayer in any case was for chemists to work on their own, reporting up the ladder, not across the aisle to other chemists. It was a style suited to industrial secrecy, and it suited Klarer. The company appreciated his talents, so they allowed him to set his own work schedule, looked the other way when he took off, and let him work all night when he needed to. Klarer made new molecules at a fantastic rate and sent them to Domagk for testing. He was the most productive chemist the company had. No one else could come close to his output. Domagk worked just as hard and just as diligently, taking the compounds mixed with certain dyes and applying them to the *Streptococcus* bacteria and summing up the results. Then the two of them together would determine the next move.

Klarer worked well with another chemist named Mietzsch. They worked in Workroom 4, tracing the patterns of atoms, unlocking the structures of chemicals, finding ways to take them apart and re-form them, altering them slightly, creating new compounds, hoping that one would become Bayer's next miracle medicine. Meanwhile, Domagk would apply their wares to the task of conquering the strep bacteria.

At first the team of Domagk and Klarer worked on finding a compound of dye and molecules that would kill *Streptococcus*. One would wonder today why they spent their time on that particular germ, since all it causes today is a sore throat, but in the 1920s and into the 1930s, it was one of the most feared killers on Earth. No one was safe from strep or staph infection.

In the summer of 1924, the son of President Calvin Coolidge got a blister on his toe while playing tennis. In a couple of days he got a fever, and an analysis of his blood showed he had an infection from *Streptococcus*. Everything that could be done was done in the days that followed, but on the seventh day from when he got the blister, he died. This is an example of how staph or strep infection could cause the least of harms to end in tragedy. It is an example of how little we knew back then about how to take effective action against the bacteria they knew were doing the damage. I felt that this description of a person with a fatal blister on his foot would demonstrate the power of this *Streptococcus* germ and why Domagk and Klarer spent so much time working on a medical cure for this deadly infection. This was the same problem that Domagk had seen in the trenches of France in 1914, twenty-four years before, and it still persisted in causing bodily harm to man—with no end in sight. Strep along with staph infections were every doctor's nightmare. These germs could be found anywhere. Remember that bacteria can lie around for years, just waiting for a chance to give man an infection. Most strains of strep were harmless, but a few were deadly, and if they got beneath the skin or in a cut, they could cause a significant number of human diseases. The worst strains of strep could secrete three poisons, wipe out red blood cells, raise fevers, eat through tissue, fight their way through the body's natural defenses, and create havoc in strong human beings. They didn't affect only the weak; they had no supranational thoughts. They just waited or hitchhiked to wherever they could find an opening. Readers who are interested in reading about these diseases should read the referenced book.

So, day after day, week after week, Domagk and Klarer fought this battle. Klarer was fantastic in finding new molecules by changing a carbon atom on the end of a string of atoms, or adding a hydroxyl to the string of atoms. Sometimes they would stay with the same dye and try combinations of different molecules; no combination affected the strep germ. Then they tried a combination of dyes while holding a molecule constant to see if the different dyes would penetrate the evil germ and carry a molecule with it, perhaps to end in a kill. But none would come. Each failure would make Domagk stay in the lab and think about what had been tried to date. He kept meticulous files on the various combinations of chemicals and dyes.

The year 1928 passed. At times they thought they had found a combination that worked, but when they tried it a second time they didn't get the same results. It gave them hope as Domagk tried to determine what had changed. It had worked the previous time; why not this time? He repeated the experiments over again and again. Finally he would send a message to Klarer to work on another combination.

The year 1929 passed, and Domagk began to think that there was no combination that would work. It was frustrating, because they believed at times that they were on the right trail and then the results they were looking for eluded them. It was fortunate that Klarer didn't lose any of his energy or run out of combinations. They say that "misery loves company"; here was misery, and he was glad that Klarer was his company. The year 1930 passed.

During 1931, their fifth year in this battle, Klarer and his partner Mietzsch were trying compound after compound. Each compound was identified with letters preceding the number, so "Kl" meant it came from Klarer and "M" meant it came from Mietzsch. They had produced hundreds of compounds, which Domagk had injected into the strep germ with little success. Every so often there would be a hint of success, only for them to find that something had given them the wrong answer. Each of these compounds found its way into the tropical-disease group to be tested there against other diseases besides the strep. Klarer investigated the use of the azo dyes with some of his compounds. Some of the azo dyes began showing activity against tropical diseases, fighting bird malaria, rat leprosy, and sleeping sickness. Finally, encouraging strep results emerged with some mice on one of the compounds, Kl-517. Like his Kl-487, it included a chlorine atom. It had a great effect on mice that had been injected with a super strep; some mice recovered completely after receiving Kl-517.

Meanwhile, Bayer remained very patient. Domagk was working on other tropical medicines on another project with some success. They were having very prosperous years as their market grew, and their profits allowed the research lab to continue their research. At times Domagk wondered how the company could be so patient when he was losing his patience, but the funds kept coming and his experiments continued.

One day Klarer's boss happened to be talking to him about how well sulfur had worked for dyeing wool some years before. This got Klarer thinking about adding sulfur as a side chain. In the first week of October 1932, Klarer delivered a compound that included a sulfur compound. The compound was noted as Kl-695. While Domagk was away, the technicians kept his program going. They noticed that the mice who received compound Kl-695 didn't die and, in fact, were running around in their cages with a great deal of energy. When he returned, Domagk reviewed the notebook that he kept, which the technicians had maintained while he was gone. As he looked down the list, there were *W*'s with double and triple plus signs, meaning they had worked well; it was nothing like Domagk had ever seen

Domagk relayed this information to Klarer and told him to try some sulfonamide with a certain dye. The next afternoon he had this mixture. Domagk couldn't believe what he was seeing in the microscope. The germ was curling up and dying. He told Klarer about the effects he was seeing, and they tried to duplicate it. Sure enough, it killed the strep. They waited a day and tried it again; the results were rapid and thorough.

Domagk decided to keep this success quiet until he tested whether this mix worked on the staph infection as well. The next day he had his mix and went to work on the staph germ. He had a hard time believing it, but he had the same results. At this time Domagk knew he had produced the secret formula. He could have patented the medicine, but he thought about the French. He feared the French and their ability to make improvements on a patent of the Germans'. Every time one of the pharmaceutical companies came up with a new medicine and took it to market, the French would copy it, improve it, and gain a bigger market share. They were better at marketing their products. So he decided to hold off. He got with Klarer and told him to try every combination of sulfur compounds with the dye. He wanted to find the very best version, so that when it was patented and introduced to the market, maximum market share and profits would result. In early 1932 when a cure was found they decided to delay and see which of the sulfur compounds gave the best results.

I am going to jump from this point in the story and cover another dilemma that was occurring during this time frame that eventually relates to this work with bacterial infections. I will bring you back to this point so as to review the progress.

## *Childbed Fever and Deaths*

Meanwhile, the British doctor who had been on the French side of the trenches was back in England working on problems that were unbelievable. Leonard Colebrook was second in command at the St. Mary's Inoculation Department in London. He was a baby doctor, not one who delivers the babies, but the one who was responsible for developing possible cures for the problems associated with the birth of children and the safe recovery of the mother throughout this ordeal. In the 1920s and early 1930s, the field of obstetrics was formed—a field made up of male doctors that were highly trained and skilled had taken the place of midwives, only to find themselves surrounded by much illness and death of the mothers and babies. Postpartum death often came in double doses, taking both the baby and the mother. Birth was looked upon as a major operation; and, worse of all, the biggest killer was the strep germ. The obstetricians could see the problem but had no defense against it.

There was a shift in the early 1900s toward mothers giving birth in hospitals instead of at home. Hospitals took over, thinking that this was the best place to have a child and thus avoid the sanitary obstacles in homes. It was much like today, when we consider the hospitals much cleaner than our homes and the major number of births in the United States is in the hospitals. The problems faced by the obstetrician in the 1920s and early 1930s related to infections that were overwhelming. Colebrook had tried Ehrlich's Salvarsan, which had been developed for syphilis, to fight the disease, with no success. Doctors were convinced by the success of Salvarsan with syphilis that there would be other diseases to be fought with chemicals. Chemicals could work against a bad disease as traumatic as syphilis, so why wouldn't it work against infection? They worked day in and day out to try and find something that would relieve the world of infant deaths at birth and the deaths of many of the mothers as well. Colebrook, like many doctors, was frustrated that the death rate for mothers had increased instead of going down. He tried everything. He had the female ward cleared of patients and the rooms scrubbed and disinfected. Bedding was burned. He took every step that should resolve any issues of death being caused by poor hygiene or other problems that might prevail in hospitals more than in homes. He stayed awake at night looking up at the ceiling and going over the various phenomena that go on in hospitals that could escalate this problem. The next day he would begin again.

Hospitals themselves had become the centers for infection by strep, rather than providing relief. Colebrook had seen this sort of thing in France during the war. Some of the routines used in the war were tried without success. Colebrook tried other arsenic compounds, remembering Ehrlich's successes with an arsenic compound, but he had the same failure. The problem was so bad and so prevalent that it had a name: "childbed fever." One out of every five new mothers died. History has shown this type of disease as far back as records have been kept, even in the time of Hippocrates in ancient Greece. Terrible bouts with this problem occurred in the seventeenth century several times.

Childbed fever led to the psychological breakdown of the doctors, who were stressed to the point of illness themselves. (77) It was frustrating to take the many precautions that they knew had not been taken by the midwives who had previously attended births at the homes of many mothers under much worse conditions than at the clean hospitals. Yet nothing worked.

By the time that Leonard Colebrook became involved in this predicament in the 1920s, childbed fever had been responsible for the deaths of tens of thousands of new mothers every year. He believed the only way to resolve the issue was through the use of chemicals. He went to Germany and spent the summer learning their language and learning about the use of chemicals for fighting diseases. By 1929 he was considered an expert in the use of chemicals to fight diseases, only to find frustration when it came to childbed fever. In 1930 he stopped giving transfusions and trying new chemicals and gave up trying to find a cure, returning to the old-fashioned approach of providing new mothers and their infants with the best nursing care and otherwise leaving them alone. He endured unbearable frustration. (47)

In 1931 Colebrook took a new position at Queen Charlotte's brand-new maternity hospital, which included a hospital-within-a hospital devoted to the isolation, care, and study of childbed fever victims. At the age of forty-eight he began this new venture and his fight against *Streptococcus*. He was committed; but so was *Streptococcus*.

I provided this background so that you will be able to relate to this terrible situation and how the progress made by Domagk and Klarer might eventually help relieve this situation. It's hard to conceive of such problems with childbirth these days ... especially at the level they were experiencing in the 1920s and early 1930s.

### Success at Last in Overcoming Disease Caused by Bacteria

Now refinement became the battle, as the team at Bayer tried to determine the right amount of sulfanilamide for injections, among other refinements. Some were stronger than Kl-695; one in particular, Kl-730, was the most effective and most consistent anti-strep medicine anyone had ever seen. They focused on Kl-730 and looked for side effects. Many drugs work, but some have side effects that are worse than the disease it cures. This labor of patience became the mode of the day. Domagk would take the mice and put a slit in their stomachs and check for problems in this area—no problems. Animals without Kl-730 died by the next day, and animals given the Kl-730 had healthy organs, healthy tissues, and no sign of *Streptococcus*. Now at the height of their exhilaration, they had to make a decision. They now knew they had a medicine that cured strep— should they patent it and allow others to see their work and copy it?

In 1935 Bayer released the new drug, called Prontosil, marketed as a cure for *Streptococcus*; it had also been successful with several other diseases, including limiting the effects of *Staphylococcus*. They claimed "remarkable effects," and the world began beating down the doors to obtain some of this miracle medicine. There was a limited supply of the medicine, mainly due to the fact that it had to be mixed properly with Bayer's azo dye. The company was purposely vague about some details because they wanted to control the market, and they were especially concerned with France.

### Enter Colebrook and the End of Childbed Fever

Sir Henry Hallett Dale, first director of England's National Institute for Medical Research, contacted Bayer and asked for samples to give to Colebrook for studies related to childbed fever. Eventually he got a message from Dr. Horlein of Bayer telling him he could have as much as he needed. Months passed before the Prontosil arrived. In January of 1936, Colebrook reported the results of almost six months of mouse testing, indicating the results were not as good as expected. He felt that he might have to do more tests before trying it on a woman. On January 6, his colleague Ronnie Hare accidentally pricked himself with a glass shard, and within two days an infection had spread throughout his bloodstream. It was doubtful he would live. Colebrook had no choice but to try the Prontosil. He gave it to him intravenously and orally. Hare turned red almost immediately and within two days was completely recovered. The first childbed fever patient that Colebrook decided to use it on was suffering from peritonitis; the strep had entered her abdominal cavity. Her pulse was racing and her temperature was rising, and it appeared she would meet the fate of so many before her. Colebrook didn't know how much to give her, so he gave her a massive dose. Within hours her fever was gone and the infection had subsided.

Colebrook felt this may have been just good fortune, but as he tried it on various new mothers he began to realize the miraculous nature of this medicine. As conservative as he was, it became obvious that the new drug worked and it worked fast with every one of the patients he gave the new drug to. (47) Colebrook and another associate, Kenny, who was involved in these tests, submitted a short paper to *The Lancet* on the success they were realizing. This was the beginning of the end of childbed fever—a miracle for mothers giving birth and for the children it helped with other medical issues.

### Then Came France and a True Find—Serendipity at Its Best

In France Ernest Fourneau, a leading French chemist, tried the same path as Colebrook, and he contacted the right people in Germany to try to obtain some Prontosil.

Eventually Fourneau received a small sample of the Prontosil and decided to do some experiments of his own. He injected forty mice with a strong dose of *Streptococcus* and then put twelve without Prontosil in a cage. He intended to inject the remaining twenty-eight with the Prontosil to determine the impact of this magic fluid. Soon after starting his experiment, he realized he might not have enough to dose the remaining twenty-eight mice. As careful as he was in parceling out the injections, after injecting twenty-four of the remaining twenty-eight, he ran out of Prontosil. He still had four mice, so he sat down and thought about what he should do. He looked around his lab; he had some sulfonamide; knowing (from people he had talked to) that the Prontosil had some amount of sulfa drug in it, so he decided to give the remaining four mice an injection of the sulfonamide. This he did, and he put them in a box and went on his way.

The next day he could hardly wait to see the results with the forty mice. He rushed to his lab and looked in the cage with the twelve mice that had received no Prontosil—there were twelve dead mice in the cage. He hurried to the second cage, and there were twenty-four mice running around with no apparent effects from the huge dose of strep they had received the day before. He was elated. Then he looked in the box to see how the four that received the sulfonamide were. To his delight, they were running around as peppy as the twenty-four that had received the Prontosil. He couldn't believe it. He decided to wait another day and visit the two cages of live mice. When he returned the next day, he was met by twenty-eight live mice, including the four that had only received sulfonamide, looking frisky and ready for some food.

Fourneau couldn't believe that the Germans had missed this simple approach. Here was serendipity; if he hadn't run out of the Prontosil, he wouldn't have tried the sulfonamide. He calmed himself and decided to do some additional tests on other mice and with the sulfonamide. This would take some time; he wanted to make sure he wasn't fooling himself. As the days went by, he became more and more impressed with the sulfonamide. There was not one failure in over a hundred tries. He kept coming back to this question:

how could sulfonamide be this effective against this deadly germ? Fourneau contacted the Pasteur Institute and arranged for them to do some tests on the sulfonamide also, and their results confirmed his results. Within three months of Domagk's publication in *The Lancet*, the Pasteur Institute began distributing their version. It was almost impossible to believe that a simple, common, unpatentable chemical that was used throughout the dye industry and on farms could be so potent a medicine, and no one knew how it worked. It was a miracle, an inexpensive miracle—the first chemical cure for a disease, Prontosil—and now simple sulfonamide. Many lives would be saved by a lot of work from the German group and a case of serendipity for the French group. And many people would benefit through the availability and low cost of sulfonamide.

The announcement by the Pasteur Institute of the results with plain sulfonamide hit the German group like a ton of bricks, and doctors around the world couldn't believe that this devil of a disease could be tamed by a common chemical. (42)

Of course Colebrook in England was elated. He began tests on his childbed fever candidates, and they were released from the hospital within days of giving birth. The average reader today may not be able to appreciate this major conquest. It was like winning a war over this deadly germ. It was like freeing women the world over from fearing death when having a child. This is one of the wonders of life.

### United States Medical Actions

One of the world's most renowned medical institutions then was (and still is today) Johns Hopkins, located in Baltimore, Maryland. They tried to get some of the Prontosil; two physicians, Perrin Long and Eleanor Bliss, intended to address various illnesses with this drug. However, they were not able to obtain any. Finally a laboratory at DuPont was able to deliver ten grams of pure sulfa to get them started, and start they did. Bliss got wonderful results with mice, and Long, based on the experience of Colebrook and his doses for childbed fever, began to work directly with patients. A seven-year-old girl with severe erysipelas, skin flaming, and a fever of 105 was treated after everything else had failed, and she was cured in days. They used it on scarlet fever, tonsillitis, and a botched abortion, with uniform success. The news from Johns Hopkins set off exhilaration around the planet. Here was another world-renowned institution, along with the Pasteur Institute and the reports from Colebrook in England, reporting nothing but great news. It was used on Franklin Delano Roosevelt, Jr., in December 1935 and January 1936. He was close to death and was saved by this medicine and became a high-profile case that helped to solidify its use in the United States.

The first official communication about the breakthrough discovery was not published until 1935, more than two years after the drug was patented by Klarer and his research partner Fritz Mietzsch. Prontosil was the first medicine ever discovered that could effectively treat a range of bacterial infections inside the body. It had a strong protective action against infections caused by streptococci, including blood infections, childbed fever, and erysipelas, and a lesser effect on infections caused by the other cocci.

Later it was discovered by a French research team at the Pasteur Institute that the drug was metabolized into two components inside the body; a smaller, colorless, active compound called sulfanilamide was released from the inactive dye portion. The discovery helped establish the concept of "bio activation" and dashed the German corporation's dreams of enormous profit, since the active molecule sulfanilamide had been first synthesized in 1906 and was widely used in the dye-making industry; its patent had since expired, and the drug was available to anyone. (77)

Of course, with every good there is always the bad. The use of sulfonamide was not to escape this bad portion of this story. Soon little labs around the United States were making their version of sulfonamide; some worked very well, but there were deaths occurring around the States. Research on the reason soon brought answers. All the deaths occurred when one supplier's medicine was used. It was determined that the problem related to the supplier using diethylene glycol (antifreeze used in cars to prevent radiator water from freezing) in his drug mixture.

As a result of this catastrophe, a federal law was passed in 1938: the Federal Food, Drug, and Cosmetic Act, which controlled how drugs would be tested and approved before their distribution for use and sale.

## World War II and the Sulfa Drug

As the most effective antibiotic drug to fight many of the diseases that a soldier can receive in a war as gigantic as World War II, the sulfa drug was untouchable. In the battles of the Pacific against the Japanese, it is believed that it played an immense part in the defeat of the Japanese. While Japanese troops were dying from infection, tropical diseases, dysentery, sexual diseases, and others, the American troops were being saved by sulfa drugs of various new combinations and released for duty in rapid order. Each soldier was ordered to carry a pouch that contained sulfa powder, to be sprinkled on wounds received on the battlefield or in accidents that occur in large numbers during war. (It's worth mentioning that the term *sulfa drug* was used instead of the bigger name. I was the recipient of sulfa for sickness in 1947 and 1949.)

The war in Europe, although less dramatic in its impact, benefited from the sulfa drugs carried by the Allied soldiers on D-Day and throughout the campaign to defeat Hitler and his army. It must have been ironic to many that its use in Germany, where the research began, helped to defeat the Germans. The pouch the Allied soldier carried with him into battle in Germany contained the antibiotic invented here.

As I mentioned, war brings bad and good things. The medical profession wanted to try some new variations on sulfa drugs, but in order to determine the results there had to be a large number of people, to provide both a control group and a medicated group. This is hard to come by, but the military provided just that. During World War I, there were many cases of meningitis, bringing a 70 percent death rate to the soldiers that fell victim to this disease. Early data from the field of war showed that new sulfa drugs, believed to be an improvement over the original sulfonamide drugs, did show definite improvement over the original. As the war proceeded, this death rate eventually dropped to 4 percent, which was an amazing statistic. (77)

During the course of the war, based on the meningitis cure rate, army doctors wanted to determine if the drug could be used to prevent the disease. Here again, large numbers of people were needed to provide a statistically meaningful sample size. It was decided to study military personnel who were going through basic training. In several cases upwards of fifteen thousand military personnel were split into groups, those who received nothing and those that took one of the pills each day, which were provided to the group that ate in one mess hall and not to the ones in the other mess hall. Over the course of several months the personnel not receiving the pill experienced forty cases of meningitis. The ones receiving the pill experienced none. Other experiments of this nature showed the same rate of response or better. It was then obvious that the drug could be given to children to prevent meningitis. By 1950, meningitis had practically disappeared from American children. Sulfa drugs were one of the wonders of life.

### A Reward for Gerhard Domagk

In 1939 Gerhard Domagk was awarded the Nobel Prize in medicine and physiology, an honor that Adolf Hitler forbade him to accept. (78) Hitler was incensed when a Nobel Peace Prize was awarded a few years earlier to an anti-Nazi activist, and he refused to acknowledge its existence. Domagk would accept the award in 1947 when the war was over. It is ironic that when he was receiving his Nobel Prize that the use of sulfa drugs had declined because disease organisms were able to mutate and began to remain unaffected by sulfa drugs. One of the main uses for sulfa drugs had been to treat gonorrhea during the war, and now it was ineffective against gonorrhea. Gerhard Domagk passed away in 1964 from an unknown disease.

### And How Did It Work?

As good as the development of Prontosil was and as fortunate as the French were to accidentally find the simple sulfonamide solution, none of them knew how it worked. Perplexingly, it had no effect at all in the test tube, exerting its antibacterial action only in live animals. This was unique in itself and still poses a problem with some of today's developments in antibiotics.

It took a couple of years for two English bacteriologists to find out how it worked and why it didn't work in the test tube. When *Streptococcus* enters the body, it attacks and consumes an enzyme, dihydropteroate synthetase (DHPS), for its nutritional needs; it swallows them up in great quantities. DHPS catalyzes the conversion of para-aminobenzoate (PAVBA) to dihydropteroate, a key step in folate synthesis. Folate is necessary for the cell to synthesize nucleic acids. (You will find that nucleic acids are essential building blocks of DNA and RNA later in your reading), and in its absence cells are unable to divide. Ironically, the sulfa drugs acted like the Trojan horse that we all read about, in that it "looked" like the enzyme mentioned above. So the strep consumed the sulfonamide instead of the enzyme and died of malnutrition, so to speak. Isn't Mother Nature wonderful, and isn't life a wonder?

### Sulfa Drug and Its Conclusion

You are probably wondering why I gave so much information on the development of sulfa drugs. There are several reasons. For one, I wanted the reader to develop a feel for the amounts of time and patience required to develop a drug such as this. I also wanted to show how fortunate one has to be to have something this difficult and compelling drop into one's lap when least expected. I also wanted the reader to see the serendipity that can be involved. It took years to get to Prontosil, and there was a French bacteriologist lucky enough to run out of Prontosil and pick up sulfonamide instead, only to find that this readily available chemical could perform like Prontosil. I also wanted the reader to have a feel for the frustration of a person like Klarer and his associate Mietzsch, who got no credit for the discovery of Prontosil. I wanted the reader to read about the first antibiotic and have a feel for the advancements in medicine and how far the world has come since then. I wanted the reader to see the ironic nature of this drug and how it helped the Allied troops in the Second World War, while being of no value to the German and the Japanese troops. I wanted the reader to see how tough childbirth was for both baby and mother not too long ago. This is a terrific story. Many of the facts came from the book *The Demon Under the Microscope*, by Thomas Hager, and from Wikipedia on medicine and sulfonamide. I considered this a marvelous example of the wonder of life. No fiction approaches the excitement of the wonder of life.

### Serendipity with a Fungus: Penicillin

I will now cover some additional serendipity (the gift of finding valuable or agreeable things not sought for; in other words, "luck") that would contribute a step to the education of many and become a wonderful aid to mankind.

In 1928, before the discovery of the sulfa drugs, a doctor from Scotland, Dr. Alexander Fleming, while practicing his art in his London laboratory, made a discovery that can be called a "super-serendipity" for the world.(43) Fleming was called "Mr. Petri Dish" because of his practice of keeping many of his bacterial experiments in shallow, saucer like dishes. In some would be *Streptococcus* and in others there might be *Staphylococcus*, each of which he worked on to try and find a chemical that would make them ineffective. On one weekend, he left for an extended holiday and didn't clean out all the saucers that were left on the windowsill of his laboratory. When he returned, he hurriedly looked over the dishes on the sills that he had forgotten to clean prior to leaving. He observed that a stray mold had grown on the outer edge of one of the saucers. He noticed that the mold had a sort of halo. When he looked at this under the microscope, there was serendipity. The mold on the edge of the saucer had killed all the *Staphylococcus* on the outer edge of the dish. Fleming viewed this mold under the microscope and noted that it was made up of very small sticklike creatures. His observations matched some prior knowledge, and he realized this was called by the name penicillin. Penicillin had been recognized many years before. Although Fleming wasn't the first to identify penicillin, he was the first to recognize the effect it had on powerful bacteria.

I have written about *Streptococcus* and its terrible effects before the introduction of the sulfa drugs, but I didn't go deeply into staph, as it is called. Staph is part of the harmful bacteria family of cocci, and, like strep, the disease they brought on did great damage to people. Remember, I mentioned that the sulfa drugs counteracted certain illnesses, but sulfa drugs were not as effective against staph infections. Staph and strep are harmful germs and under the microscope are easily distinguished one from the other, by the way they line up. Those that line up in a line like a bunch of soldiers are the strep family. These are the ones the sulfa drugs were able to overcome early in the life cycle of the sulfa drugs. Those that do not line up regularly but form groups are part of the staph family. Staph causes blood poisoning, and those with this problem were usually a short time in the world in 1928. There was not much to choose from to treat these two deadly microbes.

Of interest is the difference between mold and bacteria. They both destroy the material they live from. Bacteria in the body and throughout the air thrive in the climate of the human body. It's nice and warm and moist. Molds like moisture also, but they require the temperature of the air they live and grow in. They live in different environments, so to speak. Mold and bacteria are quite different when viewed individually under a microscope. Bacteria come from a biological group named prokaryotes. This group has no nucleus within its cells. Humans, animals, and plants come from a biological group called eukaryotes, whose cells do have a nucleus. Mold is in the latter family.

The biological families of prokaryotes and eukaryotes will be discussed in detail later in the book. I bring them to the reader's attention at this point so as raise the differences and at the same time point out some similarities between these two. It is also interesting that one affects the other, as Fleming noted during his work with mold and the deadly bacteria. Later in the book I will discuss how scientists are able to learn how mold kills the deadly bacteria in a war in the human body. (79)

Fleming discovered one problem with this serendipitous finding—the unexpected gift was not easily reproduced. In fact, as much as

Fleming wanted this unexpected gift, it tauntingly went away like a shadow at night. Try as he might, he discovered the mold was not easily found or easily reproduced. Whenever he did produce it in his broths, it would vanish while he tried to separate it. In the same building as Fleming's laboratory was another laboratory that studied such things as molds. Fleming wanted to determine the type of mold and took his mold down to their laboratory, which was under the direction of C. J. La Touche. He noted that the mold studied there was the same as one of the molds in this laboratory, and they described it as a penicillin-type mold. He felt that this laboratory may have been where the mold had originated.

Fleming worked on trying to replicate the mold and the action of the mold. His finding was that it indeed annihilated the germs he worked with, but for only a short time. He could not find a way to extend its effectiveness past thirty or so minutes. He was not a chemist and was weak on what chemical he could introduce to make it endure for a longer period. He did give a paper on the actions of this mold, but the presentation was received by a fairly uninterested crowd. He downplayed the fact that its life span was limited. It was frustrating, and eventually Fleming dropped his studies on the mold.

However, every so often, Fleming would return to penicillin, when he had an idea on how to increase its durability. After trying and failing, he went about his other business of finding solutions with other approaches. However, his interest would reach a peak every so often. He revisited his work on a solution in 1934 and then again in 1936, but with the same lack of results; but he had started something worthwhile.

### Florey the Australian and Penicillin

In 1939, Australian scientist Howard Walter Florey and a team of researchers that included Ernst Boris Chain, A. D. Gardner, Norman Heatley, M. Jennings, J. Orr-Ewing, and G. Sanders began work on trying to solve the problem of developing a method to create large viable batches of penicillin at the Sir William Dunn School of Pathology, University of Oxford, in England. (44)

It is said that Florey was an abrasive Australian who made heavy demands on his peers and the people that worked under him. This abrasiveness rarely came out, but when it did he was like a person possessed, shouting louder than those whom he confronted. It is said that he wouldn't call a spade a spade; he would call it a bloody shovel. As outspoken as he was, the people that worked with him knew it wasn't anything personal against them, and it is said he never said anything good about himself. He was very confident as well as very competent. Florey was promoted to professor of pathology at the Dunn School of Pathology. At the age of thirty-seven, Florey interviewed and accepted Ernst Boris Chain, a German Jew, eight years younger than Florey, as his chemist in the School of Pathology. He felt that in order to advance the study of pathology and biochemistry he would need a qualified man, and he got one. His next addition, in 1937, was Norman George Heatley. In 1936 Florey had assigned Chain to work on the investigation of carbohydrate metabolism of cancerous tumors. Chain felt he needed someone proficient in microdissection to effectively carve the tumors to study them. He recommended twenty-five-year-old Heatley, and after a long conversation with Florey, Heatley was brought into this technically competent group. Dr. Margaret Jennings also joined the Dunn School's staff and eventually became Florey's general assistant. She had what Florey lacked: a command of written English that was more than acceptable. For the next thirty years she would partner with Florey and present thirty technical papers.

Florey's longest and hardest search was for money. There was very little money for research of the nature he was pursuing. This continued during all the years he worked on a solution to penicillin, as well as other programs in the School of Pathology. He needed this support to keep his staff together. He finally was able to convince people in the Rockefeller Foundation to provide funds to support the people he had just added. In due time those who provided funds to Florey would be well rewarded by his accomplishments.

The work on the penicillin mold was done in a very crude manner early in the program. All initial work was done in individual Petri dishes. After a period, it was recognized that the beneficial mold they were seeking could grow to about 1.5 centimeters (about 0.6 inches) in depth, so they had dishes made with little cups in the bottom; this increased production. Afterward, Heatley had dishes made with test tubes in place of the little cups, and this worked even better. Still, this resulted in a very limited amount of the serum they were developing, and, like Fleming, they found that the penicillin gave results for a limited time period. Finally they found a chemical they could inject with penicillin that provided longer endurance. This was late in 1940, and the Germans were bombing England, as they had been for around two years. Florey and his coworkers tried to ignore the bombing, which at times caused damage to the school.

It was felt that the Germans were bombing England to soften it up for an invasion. (44) As it became more apparent that the Germans were going to invade England, Florey brought his staff together and discussed what actions they should take. They had now been having some success with the penicillin drug in vitro (in a test tube), but could not make it stay in the body long enough to bring a cure. Their only limitations were being able to make enough to provide complete results and being able to produce enough to make it a viable drug in plentiful enough quantities to introduce to the country. They didn't want to start something they couldn't finish. The reason for the meeting with his staff was to determine how to hide what they had done. They were concerned that the Germans would invade the country, and they didn't want them to have access to this drug, which looked as if it could kill almost any germ they tested it against. The decision was made to destroy their paperwork and take some of the mold and put it on each of the staff's wide smocks they wore in the laboratory. In that manner, if the Germans did invade and ended up in their lab, they could destroy what was obviously being worked on and the Germans wouldn't think the mold on their smocks represented anything but dirty smocks. They accepted the idea, and they went about dutifully keeping enough mold available in case there was an invasion. Fortunately, the British air force won the battle of the air over Britain; Hitler decided he couldn't invade England without having airspace superiority. For those readers who want to read the details of the development of this drug and how they finally were able to have it manufactured in volume, you should read the book *The Mold in Dr.*

*Florey's Coat.* (44) I have provided the reader with the areas of that book that stuck out in my memory as significant while doing my research on how penicillin made its way to the public. I wanted to bring to the reader the significant contributions made in medicine during the twentieth century, which included the sulfa drugs, penicillin, and, as you will read, the polio shots that practically eliminated this dreadful disease. They are all exciting, patient forays by committed research people to solve the mysteries of terrible diseases.

At the point where they were certain of their results and had learned a method for producing it in quantity (but still by using Petri-type dishes), the only thing that remained was to find a company that would take on the drug production and produce the drug in large enough quantities for distribution. Florey found no pharmaceutical company in England willing to take it on due to constraints of the war effort. At this point Florey decided to take the drug to the United States and see if the large pharmaceutical companies there would take on the job. By this time the United States was heavily involved in the war with Germany, Italy, and Japan, and he felt it was to their benefit to find a way to develop the drug in quantity. At this point he sought the funds to pay for a flight to the States. He made contact with people who had leverage with the pharmaceutical companies in the United States, packed his valuable molds, and flew to the States. There he provided the information for producing the mold and brought to their attention the fact that the mold passed rapidly through the body, and the biggest problem was its staying long enough to make a dramatic impact.

Six US firms took on the responsibility for developing the drug to support the war effort. Their first shot at producing the drug was to find some chemical additive to allow it to have a longer reaction in the body. An interesting point is that these firms searched the world over to find a good source of the mold that provides the penicillin. They found a moldy cantaloupe in Peoria, Illinois, that proved to be the best and highest-quality source.

Soon volume production was available but was still severely limited domestically in order to meet the war's demand. It is estimated that penicillin made a major difference in the numbers of deaths and amputations caused by infected wounds amongst Allied forces, saving an estimated 12 to 15 percent of lives. Availability was severely limited. Because of rapid renal elimination of the drug from the body, demand increased due to the need for frequent doses. Since penicillin is actively secreted in urine, with 80 percent leaving the body in almost its initial form within three to four hours, it became a common procedure to collect the urine from patients being treated so that the penicillin could be isolated and reused.

The American pharmaceutical companies worked on a method to slow down penicillin elimination. They hoped to find a molecule that could compete with penicillin for the organic acid transporter responsible for elimination, such that the transporter would preferentially secrete the competitive inhibitor. The uricosuric agent probenecid proved to be suitable. When probenecid and penicillin were concomitantly administered, probenecid competitively inhibited the elimination of penicillin, increasing its concentrations and prolonging its activity. This had a major impact on the drug's ability to eliminate the germs being fought.

The advent of mass production techniques and semisynthetic penicillin solved supply issues, and this use of probenecid declined. Probenecid is still clinically useful, however, for certain infections requiring particularly high concentrations of penicillin.

### *Florey and Chain Shared the 1945 Nobel Prize in Medicine with Fleming for this Work*

The American pharmaceutical companies soon corrected the issues of volume and longevity in the body, and forms of different penicillin were produced in volume before long. Considering that it arrived in the United States only in 1942, it soon was making a favorable impact with the troops in the later parts of the war. By 1961, pharmaceutical companies could produce upwards of six billion shots a month. The biggest problem became the same one that reduced the effectiveness of the sulfa drugs: overuse. Various bacterial mutations made penicillin ineffective for many illnesses by the late 1980s, and new medicines had to be found for fighting various infections. Bacteria mutate quickly and build defenses against the medicines that kill them. In one sense it is like Darwin's theory, when he theorizes that man and animals evolve to try to overcome weaknesses. Penicillin has since become the most widely used antibiotic to date and is still used for many gram-positive bacterial infections.

## Gram-Positive and Gram-Negative Bacterial Infections

It is interesting to know the difference between the gram-positive bacterial infections and the gram-negative infections. (46) A staining method shows whether a bacterium is gram-positive or gram-negative. This is usually the first test to determine some general information about the bacteria one is viewing. Gram-positive bacteria are those that retain a crystal violet dye during the stain process. Gram-positive bacteria appear blue or violet under a microscope, while gram-negative bacteria appear red or pink. This gram classification is empirical and provides an immediate differential identification. The bacteria that show as gram-positive have one membrane layer and include *Bacillus, Listeria, Staphylococcus, Streptococcus, Enterococcus,* and *Clostridium*. These bacteria lead to various forms of infection. Penicillin drugs were more effective than sulfa drugs in handling these diseases, although the sulfa drugs are still used for specific diseases.

The gram-negative bacteria are evident in *Salmonella* (a food poisoning); *Legionella* (sometimes called Legionnaires disease. It is contacted by inhalation of misty droplets that contain the bacteria) (80); *Escherichia coli*, a food poisoning that occurs in the lower intestine (82); acetic acid bacteria, an aerobic organism that enters the system through breathing (81) and is related to bad wine or vinegar; and others that do not cause infections. Food suppliers do tests on the products they make and ship to the grocery stores. They are particularly careful on products that come from chickens and pork. These tests are effective, but every so often warnings go out to not buy certain foods being supplied by certain grocery stores. For example, they find the meat comes from certain suppliers where something didn't check out. Some recent incidental issues related back to contaminated products such as produce that is fed to the chickens and causes the problems. In many cases cooking at high enough temperatures and for long enough times to get a recommended internal temperature of the food being cooked eliminates a potential problem. Meat thermometers work well for tracking the internal temperature of meat being cooked to ensure the meat is cooked well enough.

## Developments from Penicillin

The narrow spectrum of activity of the penicillin—that is, the diseases that penicillin was effective against and wasn't effective against—along with the poor activity of the orally active phenoxymethylpenicillin, led to the search for derivatives of penicillin that could treat a wider range of infections. (83) The first major development was ampicillin, which offered a broader spectrum of activity than either of the original penicillin compounds. Further development yielded beta-lactamase-resistant penicillin, including flucloxacillin, dicloxacillin, and methicillin. These were significant for their activity against beta-lactamase-producing bacteria species, but were ineffective against the methicillin-resistant *Staphylococcus aureus* strains that subsequently emerged.

The line of true penicillin (related to the location of the beta-lactam ring) was the antiseudomonal penicillin, such as ticarcillin and piperacillin, useful for their activity against gram-negative bacteria. However, the usefulness of the beta-lactam ring was such that related antibiotics—including the mecillinams, the carbapenems, and, most importantly, the cephalosporins—have it at the center of their structures. Many bacteria have mutated against penicillin, and bio scientists keep active in finding new derivatives of penicillin.

## Mechanism of Penicillin Action

You can watch a short online movie of penicillin killing a bacterium. A bacterium is shown, and beside it is the penicillin. The bacterium lengthens just as a cell would before dividing to make two cells where one previously existed. In this demonstration, the cell lengthens and cannot divide because the penicillin interferes with the ability to synthesize its cell wall. The bacterium lengthens until the cell wall is stretched so far that the thin cellular wall cannot withstand the osmotic pressure, and it bursts. If you remember, the sulfa drugs worked quite differently. The bacteria normally consume a certain enzyme; the sulfa drug chemically resembles the enzyme, and it is consumed instead. The bacteria essentially starve to death. It's a case of misidentification. For those who want to see how penicillin kills bacteria, visit http://www.cellsalive.com/pen.htm. (45)

## Polio and Jonas Salk

Dr. Jonas Salk did his development work on a cure for polio at the University of Pittsburgh as part of a group working on a possible vaccine for this dreaded disease. While enrolled in the school of engineering at the University of Pittsburgh, I heard of Dr. Jonas Salk and his work on a vaccine to provide immunity against polio. Later I heard they were going to provide the Salk vaccine to members of the university, and I volunteered for the shot. I remember standing in a long line that extended outside the Cathedral of Learning, the University of Pittsburgh's main building. The line progressed, and soon I was inside the main corridor of the building and advancing forward to receive the shot. I remembered that my mother had not allowed my twin brother and me to go swimming in any public swimming pools while we were growing up, because of the danger of acquiring polio. This was a true worry for all parents at the time. It had been proved that one could be infected with the polio virus while swimming in water where carriers of the virus swam. I remember these thoughts going through my mind as the line moved forward, and before I knew it, I was having a shot of Salk's vaccine injected into my arm.

President Roosevelt had been crippled by this disease as a young man and began a campaign called the March of Dimes. People would donate money to the March of Dimes to provide funds needed to fight polio. Some of that money went to the university and its virus laboratory. It was here at the University of Pittsburgh medical school in Pennsylvania that Salk developed this vaccine. Several years later, I read about his battle to provide this vaccine.

Salk had arrived at the University of Pittsburgh after working with another doctor at the University of Michigan, where they together developed the flu vaccine. Their flu vaccine proved effective, and they worked on improving its effects. Salk was receiving an annual salary at the University of Michigan of around $3,000 per annum. He was then offered the position of heading the virus research lab at the University of Pittsburgh, with an annual salary of approximately $7,100 per annum—not much when you consider the amount being paid to people of his level today. A person at his level today would be making several million dollars a year, including a bonus and any stock that came with the offer to join a company or university. Some universities provide a stock program based on any new development that is discovered while one works at the university.

Salk felt that a vaccine for polio could be developed using a dead virus. There were many people working on a vaccine against polio at the time, and none of them believed in the use of a dead virus. (46)

Salk began by injecting the live polio virus into a rhesus monkey. After the death of the monkey, he ground up the monkey's kidney, where the virus could be found in quantity, and proceeded to kill the virus with the use of chemicals. He then injected the dead virus into another rhesus monkey and waited for the monkey to develop antibodies against polio. The antibodies appeared when viewed through a microscope and gave him hope that this was the way to proceed (Kluger) (47). This may sound simple to the reader, but I am not doing justice to what Salk had to go through to get to this point. I am skimming over details for the sake of providing the reader the general idea of his approach. For the details, read the book *A Splendid Solution*, by Kluger. (47)

Salk tried several methods of delivering the dead virus to see which would create the most antibodies against the polio. This involved various chemicals to kill the virus and different fluids for carrying the dead virus so as to make it easier to provide a clean and easy-to-use vaccine. One must appreciate the fact that if one live virus was still in the serum, if it were used, it would result in a case of polio. So the method had to be very clean and very exact, and it had to provide 100 percent dead polio virus in the serum to avoid causing instead of eliminating polio.

## Salk Tried Several Methods and Eventually Settled on One

Once Salk had created what he believed was a viable vaccine, he inoculated himself and his wife and two children. They all developed antibodies against polio. This encouraged him to seek some other test subjects for the vaccine. He eventually found a school for the developmentally disabled in Pennsylvania that agreed to allow him to test his vaccine on the children of that school. This research proved to be successful, and he began to campaign for this vaccine to be accepted for tests on larger numbers of children. He couldn't convince anyone to move on this approach, because most of the doctors were against a vaccine based on dead virus. Other doctors felt that this would result in some secondary effects in the long term, even if it did work. His success while at Michigan didn't seem to pave the way for him. In addition to developing the vaccine, Salk had also determined through experiments that there were three separate forms of the polio virus. These were identified as Type I, Type II, and Type III, with the results progressively worsening from Type I, a crippling disease; to Type II, a disease that forced the victim into an iron lung for the rest of his life to allow him to breath; to death with Type III.

## 1.8 Million Children to Receive the Shot to Determine Its Value

Finally Salk's pleas were answered. Basil O'Connor, head of the National Foundation for Infantile Paralysis (later named the March of Dimes), made a decision to support a major effort that would involve 1.8 million children across the States receiving the Salk vaccine on a given day. Nine drug companies were selected to discuss the possibility of supplying the drug. Salk met with them, along with O'Connor, and they proceeded to review the steps and thoroughly went over the detailed method devised by Salk. They discussed what was required to be accepted as a supplier. Of these companies, six showed an interest. This was a huge step in ensuring there would be enough of a supply of the vaccine to handle a mass inoculation across the States. In order to prove the viability of the drug each produced, they were each required to inoculate a rhesus monkey with a shot from each lot they produced. To prove viability, each company was required to inoculate nine monkeys with vaccines from nine lots produced; all the monkeys had to show antibodies for polio and be free of polio.

As the drug companies began production and inoculation of the monkeys, plans were made to determine the effectiveness of the Salk vaccine. O'Connor felt that a responsible person had to be selected to collect and analyze the data from this field trial. It had to be a person not related to the program and one who had the capability of analyzing the large amount of data from this large field trial and providing an unbiased report on the results. Professor Tommy Francis of the University of Michigan was selected, and he eventually accepted this responsibility. Professor Francis had worked with Salk while he was at Michigan. The two of them had developed the flu vaccine.

During the mass production by the six companies selected to produce the vaccine and the testing by inoculation of nine monkeys at each firm representing nine batches produced at each company, a problem occurred. Several monkeys became sick and died from polio in various parts of the country. A rapid review of the situation and the data showed that all the monkeys had been inoculated by a single drug company. A review of the site and data at this drug company revealed that a poor filter that had been added in one of the steps in processing the vaccine was at fault.

After this was cleared up, the program was back on track to begin in full force in February of 1954. However, some supply problems occurred, and the field tests were pushed back to April 1954, just as the polio season was to begin. This delay was a disadvantage, as the team experts had wanted the vaccine to be in place a few months before the peak polio season began. But, since this massive program had begun and had so much momentum, they decided to move on with the program.

A startling event occurred when the program was about to begin. The voice of Walter Winchell, a noted news broadcaster, came across a radio station that broadcast in all the states with an urgent announcement. I will paraphrase the comments of this well-recognized and popular broadcaster, who started all his programs with "Good morning, Mr. and Mrs. America" in a loud and chipper voice.

"Good morning, Mr. and Mrs. America. Tomorrow they will be delivering one million small white caskets to all the train stations and bus stations all over the country. These caskets are for the bodies of the one million children who will die after receiving the Salk vaccine that will be injected into their little bodies."

This was shocking to Salk and to the people involved in the program. However, the huge vaccination program began anyway. Of the 1.8 million children chosen, 400,000 would receive the Salk vaccine, more than 200,000 would receive a placebo, and 1.2 million would receive nothing. All the 1.8 million-plus would be tracked to provide data on a controlled basis. Factual information from the Smithsonian Institution stated that 650,000 received the vaccine, 750,000 received placebos, and 430,000 received nothing, which adds up to a little over 1.8 million.

A form showing the name; date; address; location including address of lab, city, and state; and other data would then be forwarded to Professor Francis at the University of Michigan. At a later date, each of these children would be checked for antibodies for the three forms of polio. As well, statistics would be maintained on how many came down with polio in each of the controlled groups. The reader must keep in mind the immensity of this program. Remember in those days there were no personal computers. The early computers that were available read information hand-punched on cards; 1.8 million of these cards were coming from all over the United States.

Fourteen doctors were asked by the people heading up this program about the percentage of immunization required to prove the vaccine a success. The answers ranged from 15 to 25 percent showing the antibodies without resulting polio to consider the vaccine a success. They believed that an immunization of this percent would be significant for a disease as widespread as polio. Meanwhile, as the large program was initiated, people across the country fell into one of several categories: some were anxious, some were pessimistic, some were nervous, some were optimistic, and some thought the program would result in data that couldn't determine anything. Of course there were those pushing to cancel the program because they feared many children would die.

After several months, the day when the data would be analyzed drew near, and invitations went out from the University of Michigan to many doctors and other high-profile people across the United States, inviting them to attend a scientific meeting at Rackham Lecture Hall in Ann Arbor, Michigan, on April 12, 1955. The results of the reports on the efficacy of the poliomyelitis vaccine used in the field study sponsored by the National Foundation for Infantile Paralysis that was initiated in the spring of 1954 would be shared. Of course many members of the media would be there also. By this time, television had spread across the country since its beginning in about 1949; so many people would be watching their TVs. In addition, closed-circuit TV broadcasts would be made available to fifty-four thousand doctors across the country. Of course, Salk was to attend, along with several of his coworkers from the University of Pittsburgh; there would also be many medical dignitaries and thousands of people interested in the results, especially the parents of the children who had been inoculated.

When the day arrived and guests began arriving at the lecture hall, they saw a large stage that had been specifically built for this scientific meeting. On the stage was a large white screen for showing slides. Salk and about fourteen other dignitaries were seated in the first two rows so as to have a good view of the slides. After a few comments about the program, Dr. Thomas Francis Jr. (remember I mentioned that he had worked with Salk on a flu vaccine while they were both at the University of Michigan) was introduced to the crowd. He was responsible for collating the information being received from all the locations around the States. The crowd had been expecting to see slides and was shocked when Dr. Francis went immediately to the results. He stated that the results on the two worse types of polio were completely positive and that the results on the less dreadful phase of polio were positive but not as good as the other two more dreadful stages. The people were sort of overcome by the briefness of his report and seemed stunned into silence. Dr. Francis then stated that the Salk vaccine was a complete success. There were signs of relief in the crowd from the people who had children who had received the vaccine. Meanwhile, there were shouts of joy among the crowd, and the newspaper reporters ran to their phones. Salk, who had been expecting these results, sat quietly as he hugged his wife, who was so excited she was crying. The less positive results on the milder stage of polio were found to be due to the incorporation of Merthiolate into the vaccine by some pharmaceutical companies. Salk had never used this chemical. In fact, he had heard they were going to incorporate it into the vaccine and he violently opposed this. He was thankful that most of the companies had not included it, and this result showed how detailed he had been about what was to be done to provide this vaccine.

These data brought to a conclusion the dramatic effort by a doctor who was persistent, patient, thorough, and convinced of the eventual outcome of his research. Jonas Salk was vindicated. The dead virus approach worked and was safe for use. In 1952 before this vaccine, 57,879 cases of polio were reported in the United States; in 1961, only 1,312 American children contracted polio. In 1969, there were twenty, and in 1974 there were nine. In 1979 there was one case. The impact was just as great around the world in countries that would use the Salk vaccine. Children (and adults) could begin to swim again in public pools. Russia did not benefit at all for several years due to their inability to use the Salk vaccine, and they later used the Sabin pill, which resulted in polio being controlled in Russia.

Jonas Salk established the Salk Institute for Biological Studies in Southern California in 1962. This institute's primary objectives related to the study of genetics and molecular biology. Later it turned much of its research to finding a cure for AIDS; under the direction of Jonas Salk, this institute has done significant work in its areas of focus. Jonas Salk died in June 1995 at the age of eighty.

Here was a doctor who ignored his critics and almost single-handedly defeated the dreaded polio disease. Not only that, but he opened another door to fighting various illnesses through the use of killed viruses.

When I think of Salk, I think of the times when I was a kid and my parents wouldn't allow my twin brother and me to go to a public swimming pool because they were afraid we would get the dreaded polio disease. My mother was born crippled in her left leg and limped badly all her life. I think this made her extra-cautious about this disease. It took years for people to allow their children to go swimming in a public pool.

Another significant result of all this was that the side effects that were predicted for people taking the Salk vaccine never developed. To my knowledge, not one person was affected by any side effect of this vaccine.

One more comment about polio. I read a report that was in the paper in November 2007 that 808 people in the world had contracted polio the previous year. All of these victims lived in four countries that had never received the Salk vaccine. These countries would be given inoculations before the next polio season. Isn't that a fantastic result? Worldwide, this disease has been nearly extinguished.

## The Continued Search for the Secrets of Life

During the 1800s, the search for life and what affected life continued. The improvements in microscopes led to major breakthroughs. The various diseases discussed contributed a great deal of information and knowledge to the picture of what destroyed life, which brought biologists closer to understanding more about what they were experiencing and looking for. This was not an easy puzzle. During the 1900s, this continued to be the "carrot" that was just beyond the reach of the scientists.

Scientists puzzled over the nature of life and the work done by Gregor Mendel, which was rediscovered early in the twentieth century. The work by Thomas Hunt Morgan of Columbia University on chromosomes in 1915 reopened the subject. (88) Hunt's work on chromosomes, heredity, and what controls life became very important because he essentially proved Mendel's work. Still scientists were puzzled about what in the chromosomes dictated a person's traits. The answers were not obvious, and many were discouraged and gave up on the hunt for life's secrets. So this subject went dormant from lack of success. It reminded them of the "fountain of youth" that Ponce de Leon searched for, only to meet with failure. They felt looking for what created us—where "us" means not only human beings, but all life—would be a long, desperate search that would only end in failure.

### Work on Physics Shows Another Side of Life

Work seemed to progress in the physics of what was happening, with the works of Einstein and Bohr. Major jumps occurred in understanding how the inner parts of an atom worked. As much as we know now about the atom, it always shocks me when I realize that we didn't know that a neutron was inside the center of an atom until 1932—the year I was born. The lack of basic knowledge about the atom bothered me when I found out years later, while attending college, that they had just recently discovered this fact. I was studying to be an electrical engineer and was under the pretense that we had known this for many years, only to find it was discovered only twenty-two years before. Major advances in quantum physics were made by Einstein and Bohr and various others, and these discoveries, though not medical in nature, helped to open the eyes of those studying medicine.

Scientists thought they knew everything there was to know, and they had a hard time with quantum physics because science had always believed that every motion was continuous—that is, no breaks in the continuity of actions. If you throw a ball in the air, it goes up until it reaches a peak and begins to fall. It may, for a very minute period, slow down at the top of its motion before it comes back to earth, but this was believed to be continuous motion that could be easily explained by mathematical analysis. It shocked the scientific community to realize that atoms worked discontinuously. Things didn't just keep on flowing in a nice, even flow with quantum physics. Movement occurred in quantum jumps. The electrons inside an atom didn't move from one shell to another on a continuous basis, but leaped forward to a higher energy shell, or fell backward to a lower shell, in quantum amounts. The more that the physicists worked on this issue, the more they realized it was true; things can jump from one level to another, but nowhere in between. There was no energy level in between. In 1905, one of Einstein's papers had shown this. He received the Nobel Prize in physics in 1921 for the paper he had written some sixteen years before. It took that long for scientists to believe it. So the scientists that were working on the biology of life—including the chemists, the physicists, the biochemists, the bacteriologists, and the medical doctors—found many things to keep them busy without being bothered about failing to discover what life is and where it came from.

The dormancy on looking for the secrets of life began to loosen up in World War II. Between 1939 and 1945, there were many discoveries that brought man some tools that would allow him to make progress. The work on the atomic bomb, as deadly as it was, generated advanced knowledge of the basics of the atom and radioactive material.

The bomb contributed an important tool: radioactive material to aid in research. With this material researchers could mark a protein or various other things within the human body that would allow them to observe what happened to it within the body. It provided them a visual sort of road map. The biochemists borrowed this tool from the physicists and took responsibility for finding how the body works. Earlier I had mentioned that the scanning electron microscope was invented during the twentieth century. Here was an electronic tool that allowed the biochemists to see things magnified up to ten thousand times over what the conventional microscope was able to provide. Here was a super tool to provide a new set of eyes for scientists, and they put it to work.

# The Battle between Men's Immune System and the Mutation System of Disease

There are several bacterial diseases and several viral diseases to be considered when one relates to the battle between the ability of the disease to mutate and man's immune system's ability to remember which ones it had contacted in the past and is immune to. Let's consider the bacterial diseases caused by *Staphylococcus* and *Streptococcus* and the viral diseases such as the common cold, the flu, and measles, to mention a few. When the bacterial diseases cause a person to be sick, his body's immune system begins to build antibodies to overcome the disease. Once a person overcomes that disease, his body retains the antibodies and the person is immune to any future disease of this sort. In viral diseases a common reaction by the immune system goes into effect to produce antibodies to overcome viral diseases such as the flu. The person is immune to that given species of the flu, or measles, or cold. However, all of these viral or bacterial elements mutate into a different form that can then cause a different case of the disease. The person's immune system cannot protect against the mutations of the disease, since it has not seen that form of the disease previously and has not established immunity against it.

In some cases, such as measles, a vaccine is given to the sick individual and upon his recovery he is safe from measles for life. Of better note is to take the vaccine before one is sick, and the body's immune system will build up antibodies against measles and the person is safe from that disease for life in most cases. For a person who has had flu and is protected for life from that given species of the flu, he must receive a shot each year to protect against the new mutations of that flu. The flu bug is tough in that the mutations ride right over the body's antibodies for the past flu. The common cold is a good example where the body produces antibodies against that cold and overcomes it; however, there are many cold mutations that can cause different kinds of colds in the future. As a person gets older, he or she has experienced many of these cold mutations and is somewhat protected against getting a cold in the future. Staying away from young children carrying a new mutation can help.

It is important to note the differences between the bacterial infections and the viral infections. The bacterial element can remain active forever. It sits on a chair or inside a car or wherever. The person who had been infected and recovered has nothing to be concerned about; however, other people getting in the car or on the chair can be affected by the germ as it sits there and waits—sometimes forever. A person can take antibody medications specifically for that disease and be protected against this element of the disease. A viral infection is different. It has a very short lifetime, probably seconds before its vitality is lost. It must live on a living person to gain its nutrients from the victim. It is mainly carried in the air by people who are ill with the disease and breathe out the viral infection or sneeze and this is picked up by a person within a short distance away. So the best way to avoid catching the disease is to stay away from people breathing these diseases. Stay away from crowds where there may be many individuals sneezing or breathing out these viruses. The good thing is that viral disease cannot live on a chair or in a car before becoming inactive. The story here is that man has found antibody drugs to protect against many bacterial diseases. He has found some viral injections to protect against certain mutations of a given viral disease for life.

### Cells of Prokaryotes and Eukaryotes—the Difference is the Nucleus

With the microscope advances of the 1800s, scientists were able to see that every form of life they researched was made up of cells. This was true of plants, animals, humans, and even the bacteria and viruses. The shapes of cells are quite varied, with some, such as neurons, being long sticklike figures and some being round, like our blood cells. Cells vary in size as well as shape. A woman's eggs in her ovaries constitute the biggest cells in a human, and the man's sperm cell is the smallest. It was easy for scientists to observe some animal cells, such as a chicken egg. However, there is one commonality among man and animals that is not common in the bacteria or viruses. This returns us to the subject of prokaryotes and eukaryotes, two completely different cells, and our general way of defining forms of life.

Eukaryote is a generalization for the type of cells that humans, animals, plants, and fungi have. The word *eukaryote* is derived from the Greek, where *eu* means "true" and *karyote* means "nut," referring to the nucleus; so it means "true nucleus." The most characteristic thing about eukaryote cells is that they are made up of an outer membrane and an inner shell called the nuclear envelope, which contains the nucleus. Between these two membranes are many other compartments with many functions. The purpose of this book is to cover the generalities of such things as cells without the detail that would require another book. Therefore, I won't discuss the many things that transpire between the nucleus and these other compartments within the cell. I believe it is sufficient to say that the nucleus contains the chromosomes that contain the genetic material of life. I will cover these in a later, separate section of this book.

In contrast, the prokaryotes relate to bacteria and viruses and their cells. The word *prokaryote* is also derived from Greek; *pro* means "before" and *karyote* means "nucleus." So the word means "before nucleus." This originates from a historical standpoint, since prokaryotes were on earth before eukaryotes and they have no nucleus. It is important to realize that there were entities here on earth before man. The prokaryotes were here almost from the beginning of Earth four and a half billion years ago. Plants and animals came billions of years later. When man became educated enough and observed this difference between the cells of bacteria and those of man, he decided to call one *pro*, meaning "before," since historically the prokaryotes were here before the eukaryotes and they had this difference related to the nucleus. It's as simple as that. Prokaryotes have a single cell, whereas the eukaryotes are multicellular with nuclei.

I intend to spend most of the discussion on the cells that make up man and will only take a little time to discuss the cells of the bacteria. Both types of cells reproduce and create new cells by dividing into two cells, which divide into four cells and so on. I believe it is one of the wonders of life that there are only two types of cells in the world. When you consider the vast numbers of animals, plants, fungi, and humans here on the Earth and that they have only one type of cell while bacteria have another, that's a marvel.

## Cells of Animals, Plants, and Man

Humans have an estimated 100 trillion cells, or $10^{14}$ cells, with a typical cell size of 10 microns (25 microns equal a thousandth of an inch). A normal cell weighs approximately one thousandth of a gram. All cells come from preexisting cells, which relates to my comment on how they divide. Of course this division had to start somewhere, and that's where the discussion of life begins. Within the nucleus of the human cell (and all eukaryotes) are the chromosomes that contain the genes that determine our heredity and how each of us developed. To find out how the first cells started this whole thing in humans, plants, and animals, one has to begin with sex. When I discuss how the first cells are formed, I am not discussing how the very first cells appeared on earth. I will take a stab at that later. I am relating to the first cells of a newborn, but more specifically at the very beginning when the child-to-be is still in basic, undefined form.

## Sex and Mating: The Chromosomes

In the human case, a man has sexual intercourse with a woman. During the culmination of sexual intercourse, the man releases sperm cells in the millions. If a sperm cell makes contact with the woman's egg, fertilization of the egg occurs. Once the male sperm reaches the egg, normally no other sperm can also penetrate the egg. The woman's egg contains the equivalent of female sperm plus food to feed the embryo that has been produced and will become a male or female baby. The female has twenty-three chromosome pairs; each half of a pair is called a chromatid. Sperm also contains twenty-three chromosome pairs. The last two pairs of chromosomes (chromosome 23) determine the sex of the new embryo. The female has two X chromosomes as the last pair in her set, and the male has either two X's or an X and a Y as his last pair. These combine in the newly conceived embryo to provide a complete set of twenty-three chromosome pairs; a chromatid of the male contributes one half, and the chromatid of the female makes up the other half of each new pair. If the Y chromosome combines with the woman's chromosomes, the baby will be a boy. If the X chromosome combines with the woman's chromosomes, the baby will be a girl. Below is an illustration of the male and female chromosomes that will combine and result in a normal pregnancy.

### *Genotype Specificity* (48)

Each individual is identified by a relatively unique combination of nucleotides found in long, coiled strands of DNA, organized as chromosomes, found in a cell's nucleus. The number and arrangement of chromosomes in an organism is characteristic of that organism, and can be represented as a karyotype, which is derived by arranging the chromosomes in pairs by size. The karyotype can be used to show a difference in genetic makeup (genotype), which determines the features that a person has (phenotype). Karyotypes of various humans are shown, which a baby will have from this combination of the chromosomes between the male and female involved. (48) Humans are somewhat different than other forms of life in that they enjoy sex; their mating is a form of love, and the offspring are a product of that love.

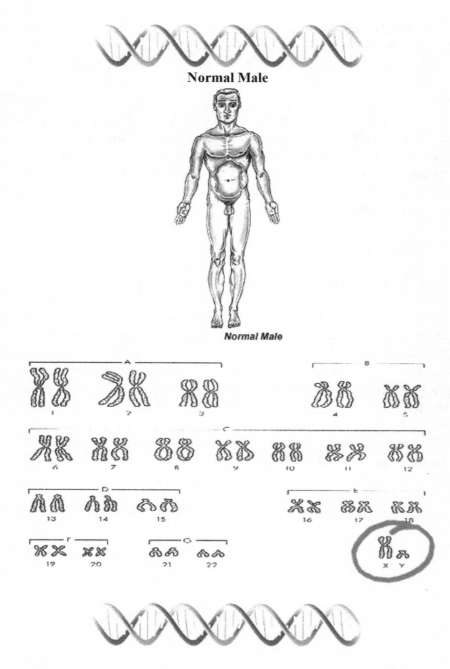

**Normal Male**

Twenty-three pairs of human male chromosomes. Twenty-two pairs are called autosomes. Autosomes determine the heredity traits of the embryo. One pair is called the sex chromosome—XY in a male. Males are associated with secondary sexual characteristics—abundant facial hair, voice, etc. Differences are also evident in the genitalia.

**Normal Female**

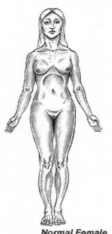

*Normal Female*

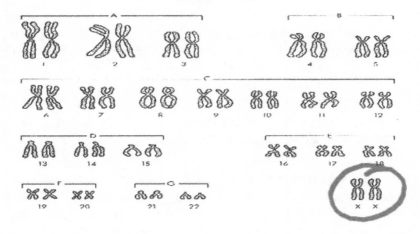

A female has twenty-three pairs as in the male, but instead, sex chromosomes are represented by XX. Female physical features differ from males. A Barr body is also present in cells of the female, representing an inactivated X chromosome.

On rare occasions, abnormalities occur as a result of certain irregularities in either the male or female chromosomes when the egg is fertilized. One such irregularity, known as *Klinefelter's syndrome*, is due to the male having a twenty-third chromosome that contains three chromosomes, including an extra Y, resulting in an XXY in the twenty-third position. This will result in a male with some breast tissue development and little body hair. An affected person is normally tall, with or without evidence of mental retardation. Males with XXXY, XXXXY, and XXXXXY karyotypes have a more severe presentation, and mental retardation is expected.

*Turner syndrome* results when a female has only an X in the twenty-third chromosome position. The second X chromosome is missing. Turner syndrome is associated with underdeveloped ovaries, short stature, a webbed or bull neck, and broad chest. Individuals are sterile and lack expected secondary sexual characteristics. Mental retardation is typically not evident.

*Down syndrome* is normally associated with three copies of chromosome number 21 (trisomy of chromosome 21), rather than the two found normally. Down syndrome is characterized by differing degrees of mental retardation, a skin fold over the eye, short stature (typically), and a short hand with a deep crease in the palm. Down syndrome is also known as mongolism.

Several other chromosomal deviations have been recognized over time, but I will not cover them in this book.

These factors had been discovered fairly early in the search for what causes heredity, and people believed in them. Still, scientists couldn't decide what determined inheritance—the characteristics of a child. They were 99 percent positive that inherited characteristics were determined by the chromosomes, but how, they didn't know. Of course they returned to the work of the monk Gregor Mendel and read through his work again and again; they reviewed the work of Hunt as mentioned. They concluded that Mendel's laws of inheritance were right, but still they sought the chief ingredient that carries inheritance. This work continued throughout the 1900s. They agreed that one parent might have the dominant hair color and the other the dominant eyes color, since these characteristics were visible, but what caused the hidden ones to be what they were? The good news, they all agreed, was that the culmination of the human sex act resulted in a human. The newborn didn't happen to have four legs like a horse—it was human.

Early in the twentieth century, the unknown elements that resulted in a child being born with certain characteristics like from his parents were called *genes*, which is derived from a Greek word that means "giving birth to." The science concerned with the manner in which genes are inherited and how the characteristics they determine are displayed was named genetics.

Late in the nineteenth century, bio scientists had begun to study, via the microscope, the cells that I have described as prokaryotes and eukaryotes. Differences were distinguishable. Eukaryotes had a nucleus, and prokaryotes did not. It was during this time that cell division was being studied by a German biologist, Walther Flemming. His studies showed that the nucleus could be observed by adding a red dye, which allowed him detailed views. This dye was called chromatin, from a Greek word for color.

During the process of cell division, he observed that the chromatin collected into pairs of threadlike bodies, which he named chromosomes because of this association with the chromatin. As he observed the splitting of the cells and the chromosomes within the nucleus, he also saw the cells line up in a threadlike position, a phase he referred to as *mitosis,* from the Greek word meaning thread. During the splitting of the cells, pairs of the cells separated, with half of each pair going to one side and forming a string of half cells (we will call this string A) and the other half of the pair going to an opposite side and forming a string of half cells (string B). This resulted in two half-cell strings—A and B—of chromosomes. These strings appear identical to the halves they came from in the original coupling that was made up of AB, and they are not identical to each other. After lining up and just before pulling apart, each half forms a replica of what previously was the half that it is now missing, which then looks like AB on one side and AB on the other side. This is called *replication*, since the original chromosome has now been replicated. When cells complete the pulling-apart phase, mitosis is complete, leaving two chromosome cells that are exactly like the original cell. How this happened was a mystery to Flemming, but he wrote about it. How the cell that split into two halves that don't look identical could then have transferred to each half the identical part each half had missed was a mystery.

This process offered an explanation for what happened during conception between man and woman with only one set of twenty-three chromosome pairs. It explained how one set of twenty-three chromosome pairs became many sets that have exactly the same genes as the original set. The genetic code had been retained and eventually produced a boy or girl, but it didn't explain how this was accomplished. One thing that was sure, when the original act of conception took place, the man only provided a sperm, the smallest of all cells in the human body. Since it had nothing in it that could contribute to any other act besides this magic mating and provide his twenty-three chromosomes, then inheritance had to be included within the chromosome pairs of the man and woman.

This became one of the big mysteries that were to be pursued for many years. Since there was only a single set of twenty-three chromosomes originally, then each of them must carry some characteristic in each of the sets. But since there are only forty-six chromosomes and there must be thousands of genes in every human body, the question was, How did these forty-six chromosomes carry all the genetics of the human body?

As the embryo that constitutes a new child grows in the mother's womb, this splitting of the chromosomes via replication and mitosis continues hundreds of thousands of times. Every cell in the body has a nucleus that contains these chromosomes, whether it is located in the arm or leg or anywhere else in the body. Remember that the adult human body has one hundred trillion ($1 \times 10^{14}$) cells. You can see that there are going to be many mitosis acts occurring over time, producing cells exactly like the originals.

Many of the scientists that were working in the 1940s on finding the genetic code for inheritance believed the chromosomes were the key. However, twenty-three could not contain all the information required for the total number of genes in a new human. Scientists believed that in order to accomplish the task that had to be carried out, each chromosome carried many thousands of genes somewhere in the nucleus of each cell. So the search was on to find the genetic information carried in the chromosomes. This search for the genes and how they performed their function was labeled genetics, and what was to follow was the search for the genetic code. Just changing the name of what they were looking for gave a great emphasis to this work. Many bio scientists in the labs that were doing research on chromosomes got excited about the name *genetic code*.

Later a Dutch botanist named Hugo de Vries was to show that inheritance doesn't always proceed smoothly. There are strange characteristics that appear every so often. He called this *mutation*, from the Latin word that meant change. Earlier I gave examples of issues in children due to a missing or extra chromosome. These are only a few of the recognized mutations, if you will. De Vries felt there were too many replications and mitosis events within the body, as well as many outside events, that could cause a change, even slightly, that results in mutations in the genes that must be within the chromosomes. Time was to prove he was correct.

Studies showed that chromosomes were very delicate and could be affected by heat, radiation, and even by vibration. It is a wonder of life that something so delicate would find a home here on earth, where there are solid forms of matter that can take all kinds of punishment without any variation. Here, the problem was just the opposite, and their fragility made it difficult for the scientists and bio scientists that worked with these fine, delicate forms of life.

## Organics, Proteins, and Nucleic Acid

Much earlier in the evolution of biology, it was determined that there were organic substances and inorganic substances. At the time all organic substances fell into one of three categories: carbohydrates (e.g., sugars and starches), lipids (oil and butter), and proteins (gelatin and egg whites). Early research focused on the proteins, the most complex of these three organics, which appear in the body in many places. Proteins were complex and fragile and appeared related to discoveries in the study of the chromosomes. It didn't take much of an argument to convince biologists and bio scientists that protein must be the thing that makes up the source of life. Because they were the biggest of the organic molecules, logic dictated that proteins would be responsible for determining the inherited factors. A protein can become denatured—unable to carry out its tasks—with heat, acids, bases, vibration, and other things that can snuff out delicate life. The chromosomes and all the work done on them showed that they were definitely delicate organic substances. Further investigation of chromosomes showed they were mainly made up of water and proteins. Since the name *protein* means "of first importance," why wouldn't it be first in importance relative to carrying the inheritance of the human race forward?

However, in 1869, Friedrich Miescher isolated a substance from tissue that was not carbohydrate, lipid, or protein. Since he had recovered it from the nucleus of a cell, he called it nucleic acid, due to its acidic nature. (50) At the time of his discovery it was not considered a major finding. Who cares that some scientist happened to find something that was not one of the three organic families? The discovery of nucleic acid lay dormant for many years. Eventually, many years later, the answer would come for his findings. This substance was found to be joined to the protein of the chromosomes and was given the name *nucleoprotein*. I will cover nucleoproteins in a later section of this book. The work of Miescher would be appreciated many years later.

A considerable time passed without any major contributions to solving how the chromosomes worked and from where we inherit our characteristics. Many of the scientists and doctors were tied up with the fighting for the life of man during the first thirty-odd years of the twentieth century. I described the major issues—plagues, flus, smallpox, infection, and wars that we were involved in—and how they each sapped man's time for doing studies on other things, like chromosomes. These problems sapped not only their time, but, in many cases, the actual lives of many of the people that would have been involved in further research. And so time passed without much in the way of advancement on this search.

## A Virus to Show the Way

An odd occurrence in 1935 started providing new clues into how nature worked. American biochemist Wendell M. Stanley isolated the tobacco mosaic virus. This virus caused a disease that affected the tobacco leaf. His studies showed the virus to be crystals that were protein in nature. This virus was not composed of cells, but rather was a fragment no larger than a chromosome. The comparison that Stanley made related to the ability of this virus to duplicate itself once it got inside the cell of the tobacco leaf—the same capability as the chromosome. This virus was also like the chromosome in that it was protein in nature, and it contained nucleic acid as well. It was therefore what was previously described by Miescher as a nucleoprotein. This finding would be followed by more discoveries over the next few years. All viruses were found to be protein and to have nucleic acid as part of their makeup. Thus chromosomes within a cell and these viruses outside the cell were shown to replicate themselves in exactly the same manner and were nucleoproteins. This gave direction to the scientific community at a time when their energies should have been directed toward the study of nucleoproteins as the possible answer to what caused life. Up until this tobacco virus was found, the direction of energy was focused on proteins. Now the focus of discovery would be nucleoproteins.

## Nucleoproteins

However, as the biochemists studied the nucleoproteins, their main focus returned to the proteins, since the nucleic portions were rather straightforward and the proteins were very complex. Take for instance hemoglobin, which was not even all protein. The globin portion was a protein, and the hemi portion was a form of iron that is in the blood to take on oxygen. This molecule was large and rather complex, but it could be split and was easy to work with. There were many other proteins that the body can take in and chemically deal with, without problems, but those proteins did not react the same way in a test tube outside the body. Not being able to study these proteins in a test tube had bio scientists looking for why. Further study found that the body deals with this issue in a different way. They found that enzymes make reactions occur readily with the proteins taken into the body.

An enzyme is a catalyst that speeds up a chemical reaction within the body. I like one of the examples that Isaac Asimov gives in one of his books. He relates enzymes to the fact that when one wants to tie his shoelaces, he bends over; it takes an effort to get this done. However, if you put your foot on a stool, it is quite easy to tie the laces. In this example Asimov says that the stool acts like an enzyme, in that it allows the process to proceed more easily and faster. When you are done, the stool looks just like it did before the procedure. This is how an enzyme works—allowing the action to be accomplished more easily and faster, without the enzyme changing during or after the process is completed. The body has an enzyme for every one of these complex actions. The unusual thing about an enzyme is that it works for one thing and nothing else. As many complex proteins that exist and are taken into the body, there are that many specific enzymes to provide the action required, and no other. Each reaction has its own enzyme, and every enzyme is a protein, a different protein than the one it facilitates. This phenomenon became known as "an enzyme for every protein."

Therefore, it is almost impossible to re-create the actions outside the body that happen in the body. This is true for all living things, not just humans. In fact, some of the same enzymes exist in a horse or pig that exists in a man, helping speed up the actions in the processing of proteins. Some children are born with an enzyme deficiency of one type or another, and they have difficult times doing things that are simple for the average child. They can be helped if the diagnosis is able to determine which enzyme is deficient and if that enzyme is provided to the child with the deficiency. In time, bio scientists would discover how to synthesize many of the enzymes and re-create the action as the body does.

To give you an idea of the catalytic action of enzymes and how fast they accelerate chemical reactions in the body, we only have to look at the reaction of orotate decarboxylase as an example. Without the enzyme, it would take seventy-eight million years to complete the reaction—with the enzyme, it takes eighteen milliseconds (eighteen thousandths of a second). Isn't nature wonderful?

There are other sources of proteins that come from outside the body and invade the body. Whenever there is a strange source that enters the body, the body considers it an invader and treats it as an antigen. An antigen is an invader of the body. When the body recognizes an antigen, it goes into action to protect the body. It forms antibodies. These antibodies are man's early protection system. It turns out that antibodies are proteins that come from the white blood cells of the body and act just as the enzymes work; antibodies can only work against one foreign protein that happens to invade the body.

At times the body and its first line of defense are not sufficient to overcome an antigen, and a doctor will provide a medical solution to the problem. In many cases the medical world has developed vaccines that protect us before the invader arrives. The purpose of the vaccine is to have the body develop antibodies specifically for a given antigen (or disease). If that antigen tries to invade the body, the immune system has already developed the antibodies to combat the invader. However, an antibody can only work against one particular antigen. If a person gets a flu shot, the body generates antibodies against the strain of flu for which the shot was developed. If a different strain of flu happens to hit the person, the antibodies will not protect him or her against that strain of flu.

This is why each year biochemists have to develop a different flu shot than the year before. Each year the World Health Organization (WHO) determines which strains of virus are reaching parts of Asia at a certain time of the year, and then they develop a flu shot that will encourage antibodies against that particular strain of flu. When it reaches North America, we are prepared for it. We are fortunate in this country that this is found out early enough in the cycle of flu to allow us to develop a specific flu shot before it hits the United States, Canada, and other countries of the world. The development of the flu vaccine is not a quick process. A culture must be prepared and put in chicken eggs six months ahead of time to allow the virus to develop prior to being useful in this yearly cycle. Just to supply the United States, this has to be done in over one hundred million eggs each year.

## Understand the Very Small Things in Our Body or Those that Affect the Body and the Genetic Code

I am spending considerable time on the subject of proteins to give the reader an idea of the extent of the number of proteins in the body, including the number of enzyme proteins, antibody proteins, nucleoproteins, and normal proteins. There are millions of them. I want each reader to get a feel for the extent of the problem that scientists were faced with when they tried to narrow down the elements that might be involved in the creation of life. The genetic code was the end result being sought by the scientists. The genetic code was like the Holy Grail that was sought many years before. What is it that allows characteristics to be carried on from one generation to the next generation and to the generations that follow? What is the secret miracle in the body that has brought us from the several humans and several animals that existed only about ten thousand years ago to this period in time, when there are over 7.3 billion humans on earth and more animals by far than the number of humans? What is it that allows us to breed dogs that are almost exactly alike—except for maybe a little different personality? When we want a German shepherd dog that is exactly like thousands of German shepherd dogs before it and has the same mannerisms that are considered a part of this species, we can get one. It turns out that each living being, whether human, animal, or plant, has its own particular species of proteins, enzymes, and antibodies and specific reactions to various invaders. This is what was being sought for the last 150 years; since around the beginning of the nineteenth century. This is one of the wonders of life that we so diligently sought. When one thinks of this complexity and trying to find what causes the results we see, doctors and scientists were almost certain that it was the proteins that determined the genetic code. They believed it had to be something with a significant number of sources, like the large number of proteins known at the time.

## *Man's Problems to Solve: The Genes And The Search For The Genetic Code*

Among all the creatures, plant life, bacteria, and viruses, only man is capable of determining the answer to this puzzle. While man is best suited for this task, it wasn't until recently that he became educated enough in life's sciences and life's mysteries to approach the answer. Equipment became available that would allow him to take steps that couldn't be taken before. When one considers that through the 1800s we didn't know what made up all the elements and didn't know there was such a thing as an atom, let alone what constitutes an atom, it's a wonder we got as far as we did.

Work was performed by chemists on molecules during the 1800s and during the first twenty or twenty-five years of the twentieth century. The atom was first described in one of Einstein's four magnificent papers in 1904. It took another twenty years or so before it became clearer how an atom's electrons spin about the center of the atom and then how they jump quantum leaps to go from one energy level to another. It took till 1932 before the neutron was discovered in the center of the atom. Physicists had data showing that there was something there, but it took many years to determine what it was. So, when one takes that ignorance into account, one can readily see why it took so long to decipher where genes came from and how they performed their magic. Keep in mind that there were no lightbulbs in most of these labs till after the nineteenth century. Likewise, there were no bulbs in microscopes till Edison invented the lightbulb. In addition, microscopes had taken us to their limit of magnifying 270 times the size. It wasn't until fifty years later that a commercial scanning electron microscope was available that allowed scientists to see some of what I am discussing.

The chemists had done a wonderful job working with molecules and staining them so they could be observed in the limited light a candle or oil lamp would provide. The chemists, biologists, medical doctors, physicists, and engineers of the time did a fantastic job of carrying the technology as far as possible without many modern tools. But time and man's persistence led to an understanding of and solution for many of these problems.

Now, just as the early scientists before us, we will continue on the trail of the genes and the genetic code.

## *Thomas Edison*

I felt that I should bring Thomas Edison's name into this writing since he contributed several things that would help scientists and doctors and all the people in the world. Around 1877, as a fairly young inventor, Edison invented the phonograph. This was just the start of an advance in communication. Now someone could make music on a record and listen to it for months. The first ones he made didn't last long. I believe they were made on a thin piece of tin. Later he improved this, adding a wax coating to a cardboard-type material. People couldn't get over this ability to hear sound from a piece of material, although it was crude relative to what was to follow. This invention set the stage for many happy times for people over the years. Here was an invention that was practical for certain applications and marvelous for entertainment as the years passed.

As important as the phonograph was, the big hit for Edison and the world was the lightbulb. Others had actually invented the basics of a lightbulb before Edison, but their approaches resulted in novelties. Earlier versions worked for a couple of hours before burning out, and they were expensive. Only the rich had them, and they used them like a novelty. But after many hours of work, Edison came up with a high-resistance filament made of carbon that worked for several hundred hours. Later he was to make production lightbulbs, using an improved vacuum and a better filament that lasted for fifteen hundred hours. I don't know if he was the one who eventually came up with the tungsten filament, but if he didn't do it, he at least set the stage for it.

Edison wasn't just an inventor, he was a production addict. He tried to find ways to produce things in high volume so costs went down and prices went down, so many people could use these inventions. Can you imagine what life was like when it was dark outside and the only light was an oil lamp or candle inside the house? Compare this to what we have now. There is light anytime that we want it. The first town that had streetlights was Menlo Park in New Jersey; Edison was the producer.

What about microscopes? Can you imagine looking at things under a microscope using only a candle off to the side? We owe a lot to the engineers and scientists that have helped to make the world a better place to live in. If we so desired, it could be void of wars.

It took men like Edison to provide bio scientists another tool to help them on their way. One thing we can say about the twentieth century: it was a great century for discovery. I could write a book about the discoveries during the twentieth century, but I only bring this to this book as a reminder for those of you scientists, engineers, biologists, medical doctors, biochemists, and bio scientists to keep working on your science, since it brings more weapons to the people that work on the elements that make up our lives.

## Amino Acids

Early in the 1800s, a French chemist named H. Braconnot heated a protein gelatin in acid and obtained crystals of a sweet-tasting compound. Eventually, this was given the name *glycine*, from the Greek word meaning sweet. (49) The structure of the glycine molecule was mapped out, and it proved to be simple. Eventually it was determined to have ten atoms, less than half the number in glucose. The molecule consists of a central carbon atom, which is attached by one bond to an amine group and by a second bond to a carboxylic acid group. The remaining two bonds are occupied by hydrogen atoms. This was eventually called an amino acid. Braconnot went further and obtained a second amino acid that he called *leucine*, from the Greek word for white, because of the crystal's color. Additional amino acids were found as the years passed, and in 1935, a new and important amino acid was discovered after a protein molecule was broken down by heat and acid. This special amino acid is called *cystine,* and you will see why it was so important.

It was determined that amino acids were the building blocks of the protein molecules. Additional amino acids were found, but as far as the biochemists—in their search for what makes up the proteins that they see relative to the chromosomes in the nucleus of the cell—were concerned, there were special ones. These special ones, Cystine, were found in every protein and added up to twenty-one known amino acids at the time. However, another one was found that was only in one protein, so this made twenty-two amino acids that related to the makeup of the various proteins. The body has twenty natural amino acids and two additional ones have to come from the food one eats. At this point in time there was no other macromolecule found or synthesized that was made up of so many different units. This discovery of the ability of the amino acids to build the various proteins is like finding a brick with which one could build a house. The brick stays the same, but the house can look completely different from all the other houses you look at, even if it is made with the same brick. This finding during the time leading up to World War II was fruitful in establishing what the biochemists and bio scientists thought was one stage of the building block of life.

I am going to briefly discuss the atomic structure of an amino acid and then provide information on how the twenty-two amino acids provide different connections to the proteins that the biochemists were interested in. Don't get nervous! The information will be supplied in a simple and easy to understand way, even if the reader is scared of trying to understand atomic structures. Think of it like putting together one of those puzzles that young children and some older people do for fun. They take the small parts and find out how to put them together to make a finished puzzle.

Remember, at that time in history, it was felt that proteins were the key to what determines genes and the inherited characteristics provided by the genetic code. As you will see, the amino acids were rather simple, and their lack of complexity, plus the large number of proteins that could be constructed from them, led many biochemists to believe they were the key to the proteins and the key to the genetic code. Shown in figure 1 below is Cystine, the foundation of the amino acids. (49) As you can see by its atomic structure, this amino acid is made up of a central carbon atom, called the alpha carbon, and it is tied to the amine group of nitrogen and two hydrogen atoms on the left and to the carboxylic acid group shown attached to the carbon atom on the right. Notice that there is an "R" connected to the bottom of the alpha carbon. This "R" represents the side chains that can be attached at this position to give the twenty-one other amino acids besides Cystine. So every amino acid has Cystine as its base. What attaches in the "R" position makes up the twenty-one other amino acids. Simple, right?

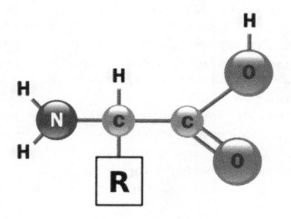

Figure 1. Cystine

The general structure of an alpha amino acid, with the amino group on the left and the carboxyl group on the right. Note: where the R is placed relates to where the twenty-one other side chains would be placed to determine the full complement of the amino acids that become the building blocks to fabricate all proteins.

You can see how simply this amino group is built up with the side chains. Each of these twenty-two amino acids, as a result of these side chains, can be part of a multiple number of proteins. With the twenty two amino acids and the large number of proteins, the combinations could form over forty thousand different proteins. This gave the bio scientists a stronger feeling that, with large number of different selections to choose from, the amino acids must be where the genetic code was stored.

## *The Magic Paper*

The story of how many of these amino acids were discovered is interesting. In 1944, a sheet of absorbent paper came to the rescue. In that year two English biochemists, A. J. P. Martin and R. L. M. Synge, devised a technique in which a mixture of amino acids, obtained by breaking down a particular protein molecule, were placed on porous filter paper and allowed to dry there. The edge of the paper was then dipped into an organic liquid that slowly moved up through the fibers by capillary action. As the liquid passed the dried area of mixed amino acids, these amino acids found themselves pulled along. Each amino acid was pulled at a different rate, and before long, each had been separated from all the others. In other words, the paper supplied a map showing what amino acids were present in the liquid being reviewed. Methods were easily devised thereafter for identifying each amino acid as it took up a characteristic position on the sheet of paper and for estimating the relative quantity of each. This was a simple but dramatic method for looking at various materials to determine the mix and strength of each amino acid present in the material being analyzed.

This technique, *paper chromatography*, for the first time made possible accurate identification of all amino acids in a particular protein. This was the first stage of the solution to the problem of finding amino acids. Through the late 1940s and thereafter, many exact identifications of the amino acids in one protein or another were performed. Martin and Synge were awarded the 1952 Nobel Prize in chemistry.

As soon as the Martin-Synge technique had been developed, another British biochemist, Frederick Sanger, solved the problem of amino-acid order. (50) His method of attack was to only break down the protein molecule partway. Instead of reducing it to individual amino acids, he stopped at short lengths of peptides, each containing no more than two or three amino acids. He separated these small peptides by paper chromatography, isolated each, and worked on it separately. Carefully, he worked out the exact order of the amino acids in each of these small peptide chains and then slowly deduced the manner in which all the amino acids must have been fitted together in long chains so that, when the latter were broken down, just those small peptides that he had detected would be produced, and no others. By 1953 he had worked out the complete amino acid order of a protein molecule called *insulin*, a hormone formed by certain cells in the pancreas. It controls the body's breakdown of sugar for energy; its deficiency results in sugar diabetes. Further work with animals determined that insulin supplied from pigs and cattle could be administered to people suffering from sugar diabetes.

This is one of the wonders of life that I am writing about. Isn't this exciting that a person could have the diligence and patience to work long and hard on something and use a piece of paper to provide him much of the answer? Do you realize how long it would have taken to find this answer without that little piece of paper and a person creative enough to invent this process and another creative enough to work out all the amino acids and discover one that saves many lives, year in and year out? It not only saves lives, it makes life bearable for many people in the world with sugar diabetes.

The American biochemist Vincent du Vigneaud used Sanger's methods to work out the exact structure of two other protein molecules, called oxytocin and vasopressin. (50)

Oxytocin is a hormone produced by the hypothalamus (part of the brain) and stored in the pituitary gland. It is used to help start or strengthen labor in a woman during birth and to reduce bleeding after delivery.

Vasopressin is a man-made form of an antidiuretic hormone. Vasopressin is normally secreted by the pituitary gland. In the body, vasopressin acts on the kidneys and blood vessels. It is used to treat *diabetes insipidus,* which is caused by a lack of this naturally occurring hormone. Diabetes insipidus is a disorder in males that causes them to urinate frequently. Vasopressin taken by affected people allows them to retain their urine longer and makes life more comfortable for them.

These two protein molecules turned out to be rather simple molecules, and du Vigneaud was therefore able to put together amino acids in the order he had deduced from his experiments. In that way, he was able to produce synthetic molecules that possessed all the properties and performed all the functions of the natural proteins. This was the strongest proof of the correctness of the theories of protein structure that had been developed from Fischer onward. This was so dramatic that du Vigneaud was awarded the Nobel Prize in chemistry in 1955, the very year of his discovery; Sanger had to wait three more years for the reward for his more general labors. It is amazing that by changing only two side chains, two completely different hormones were produced that worked on two completely different functions in the body.

To give you another example; the hemoglobin molecule contains 547 amino acids, distributed among four polypeptide chains held together by electrical attraction and by disulfide links. There are three types of hemoglobin: type A, type S, and type C. Type A is normal; people with type A with C or S will live a normal life. Those who can only manufacture type C or S will not survive long. The difference is that normal blood has glutamine; if the glutamine happens to be replaced by a valine or a lysine to make type S or C respectively, then survival is not likely. This demonstrates that where only one amino acid out of 547 is wrong, results will be a major problem.

The number of proteins the twenty-two amino acids can form according to where they are located in the given molecule turns out to be an almost infinite number. This discovery gave rise to a question: do the proteins or amino acids or a combination of these determine heredity? The larger the number, the more complex the problem of how genes can control the proper combinations and locations becomes. Maybe it isn't the proteins. Maybe it isn't the combination of amino acids, peptides, and proteins that determines heredity.

Keep in mind that out of 40,320 possible vasopressin combinations, the body chooses just one. Out of eight octillion (1 x $10^{18}$) possible combinations for one of the insulin polypeptides, the body chooses just one. How can that be controlled? We are talking about probabilities. The probabilities decrease as the number of possibilities goes up; and we are only discussing insulin and vasopressin here. What about all the other proteins and hormones that seem to beat all these odds? When one considers how many people are born and have been born since the first couple was around, and that, in most cases, they came out fine and normal, what are the probabilities for this to be so if the number of choices for failure is so high? So bio scientists started thinking that there must be instructions coming from the chromosomes' nucleus. However, how does this take place? All it takes for scientists to get excited is to tell them there is a genetic code that determines heredity, and they can't wait to experiment and find out why. Here they were, searching for the wonders of life, and they have seen how complex materials can be made of twenty-two amino acids in one combination or another.

## It Isn't the Proteins

Scientists the world over continued their research into these complex subjects, still trying to determine if the key to inherited characteristics was the proteins, the amino acids, or some combination. The answer had been there waiting, so it seems now. Pneumonia-causing bacteria come in two strains: one smooth and called S, the other rough and called R. In 1928 it was reported that a batch of S bacteria killed by boiling could be added to living R bacteria to bring about the production of live S bacteria. It was guessed that the S bacteria contained a gene that controlled an enzyme that was responsible for the smooth surface and that this was still active and changed the R (rough) bacteria to S (smooth). They felt that there was something in the S bacteria that chemically replaced what had been missing in the boiled R bacteria and converted it back to its original properties.

In 1944 this experiment was repeated when three biochemists working at the Rockefeller Institute—Oswald T. Avery, Colin M.

MacLeod, and Maclin McCarty—were able to show that the gene was in the solution of nucleic acid, without any protein involved in the experiment. [50] Other experiments were performed using nucleic acid, and the results pointed definitively toward the nucleic acid as containing the genetic code. The bio scientists were confused by this situation. How could nucleic acid hold the key to heredity?

After so many years of research on how proteins determine the genetics of a person, the sudden shift from "It's the proteins" to "Maybe it isn't the proteins" was like a truck hitting a brick wall. That's how fast the pursuit of proteins came to a halt when these three men from the Rockefeller Institute provided their findings.

Now came a quest for what was in the nucleic acid that might be the key to the genetic code. Study of the history of nucleic acid began in 1919 by a Russian-born American.

**Important – readers that have difficulty with chemistry or biology may find the following (approximately twenty-five) pages on DNA too difficult to understand. If so, go on to proceed past this section and continue reading since the material beyond that is not this difficult. I have made the DNA as simple as I can—sorry.**

### DNA and RNA

We have to go back in history to 1919, when Russian-born American biochemist Phoebus A. T. Levene first identified ribose as a component of nucleic acid. (50) Later Levene discovered that not all nucleic acid contained ribose, which is a sugar, but some had another sugar that was only different because it didn't have an oxygen atom in the molecule. He named this type *deoxyribose acid*, where "deoxy" meant "without oxygen." Over time biochemists started calling them RNA for ribonucleic acid and DNA for deoxyribonucleic acid. These two are the only nucleic acids that contain a sugar.

Further investigation showed that DNA was only found in the chromosomes' nucleus and nowhere else in the body. Most of the

RNA is found in the chromosomes just outside the nucleus. Every cell tested showed this to be true. Further investigation showed that human chromosomes had RNA both inside and outside the nucleus and the DNA was just inside the nucleus. This led to their reviewing the tobacco mosaic virus's makeup once more. It was found that the tobacco mosaic virus only had RNA.

Previous data had shown that nucleic acid is an acid because it contains phosphorus. Some proteins were known to contain some phosphorus, but nucleic acid contained 9 percent phosphorus, which is about three times the amount found in the white of an egg. This made it fairly heavily acidic.

Now we know that DNA and RNA are made up of acids—courtesy of their phosphorus content—and sugars, through the ribose or deoxyribose content. There is more to it than just the sugar and acid contents. (51)

## DNA

DNA uses deoxyribonucleic acid as its sugar. Each nucleotide consists of a nitrogenous base, deoxy sugar, and a phosphate acid.

Next it was found that DNA contained a base pair of *purines* (pronounced pure-eens) that are acids and a base pair of *pyrimidines* (pie-rim-a-deens) that are acids.

The purines are made up of a class of double-ringed chemical structures. One ring is made up of a six-sided hexagon, and the other ring is made up of a five-sided pentagon sharing one side of the six-ringed structure; there are two purines, *adenine* (add-a-neen) (A) and *guanine* (gwa-neen) (G). These are shown below in figure 2

The pyrimidines are made up of a single ring of six sides in the form of a hexagon. There are two pyrimidines—*cytosine* (si-toe-seen) (C) and *thymine* (thi-meen) (T)—they are shown below in figure 3.

A purine is only complementary with a pyrimidine. By this I mean that a purine such as adenine (A) or guanine (G) must be connected to a pyrimidine (C) or (T). This is called *complementary base pairing.*

To make things easier, biochemists started to refer to them only by their first letter and used capitals. So the allowed paired connections for DNA are A to C or A to T, or G to C or G to T. These connections can all be in the reverse order; for example, A to C could be C to A. In complementary bonding there is always the big double-ringed structure tied to the smaller single-ringed six-sided structure of the pair through hydrogen bonding. These are shown in figures 3 and 4 below.

### Hydrogen Bonding and Stability

Figure 3 shows a GC base pair, purine (G) hydrogen bonding to pyrimidine (C) through three hydrogen bonds.

Figure 4 shows an AT (adenine and thymine) base pair, demonstrating two hydrogen bonds connecting the purine A to the pyrimidine T.

Hydrogen bonding is the chemical mechanism that underlies the base-pairing rules described above. Appropriate geometrical correspondence of hydrogen-bond donors and acceptors allows only the "right" pairs to form stably. The GC base pair has three hydrogen bonds, as shown in figure 2, whereas the AT base pair has only two, as shown in figure 3; as a consequence, the GC pair is more stable.

Paired DNA and RNA molecules are comparatively stable at room temperature, but the two nucleotide strands will separate above the melting point, which is determined by the length of the molecules, the extent of mispairing (if any), and the GC content. Higher GC content results in higher melting temperatures. (51)

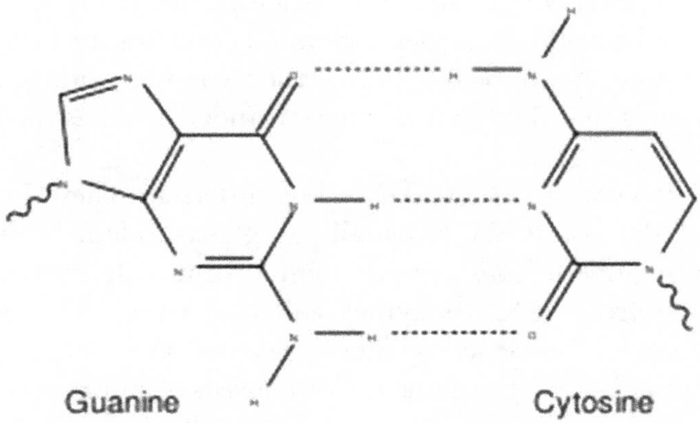

Figure 2. Base pair GC

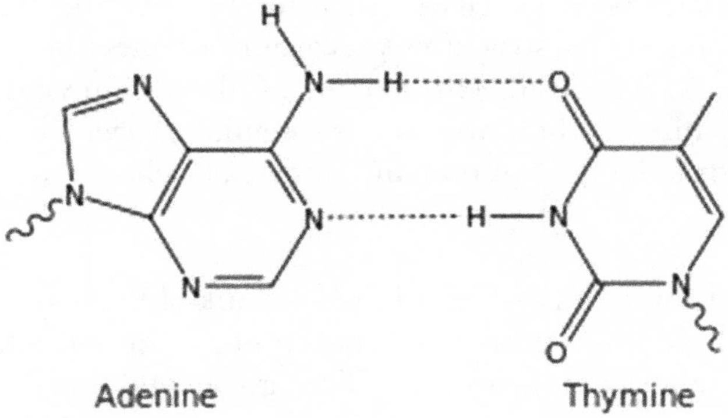

Figure 3. Base pair AT

## RNA

Ribonucleic acid, or RNA, is a nucleic acid. RNA nucleotides contain ribose as their sugar. RNA uses the uracil base in its composition instead of thymine, which is present in DNA. So if you review the base pairing shown above for DNA, and specifically the one containing thymine (figure 4), if you were looking at RNA the uracil would be in the position of the thymine with everything else remaining like DNA. So, instead of GCAT as the nucleotides of DNA there would be GCAU for the RNA, with the U replacing the T of the DNA. Uracil looks exactly like thymine. DNA is inside the nucleus and never comes out of the nucleus, while the RNA is single-stranded and outside the nucleus, so uracil performs the task in place of the thymine. As we review this further, you will understand how important it is that the RNA is single-stranded and has the uracil.

RNA is very similar to DNA but differs in a few important structural details. RNA is usually single-stranded, while DNA is double-stranded. This is a very important difference. RNA is transcribed from DNA enzymes called *RNA polymerases* and is generally further processed by other enzymes, some of them guided by noncoding RNAs. Each nucleotide consists of a nitrogenous base, a ribose sugar, and phosphate acid. RNA plays several important roles in the processes of translating genetic information from deoxyribonucleic acid (DNA) into proteins. One type of RNA acts as a messenger between DNA inside the nucleus and the protein synthesis completed in structures known as ribosomes that are located outside the nucleus in the chromosome. Others form vital portions of the structure of ribosomes, act as essential carrier molecules for amino acids to be used in protein synthesis, or change which genes are active.

When I think of DNA and RNA, I think of the ways that bees or ants behave. In each there is a queen bee or queen ant, and the other bees or ants are the workers. They go out and find food for the queen. So they are in and out of the hive or anthill on a continual basis. You will see that this is the modus operandi of DNA and RNA. The DNA is like the queen who stays in the hive (in this case the nucleus inside the chromosome), and the RNA is like the working bees moving in and out of the nucleus and doing something at the DNA's instructions. You will soon see how this works in the cells of a human. This analogy may help you to envision the methodology of the DNA/RNA actions.

Austrian-American biochemist Erwin Chargaff broke up the DNA molecule until all the purines and pyrimidines were loose. (50) He then analyzed the mixture of the two purines (adenine and guanine) and the two pyrimidines (cytosine and thymine) to see how much there was of each. In 1948 he showed that in the entire DNA tested, the total number of purine molecules was always equal to the total number of pyrimidine molecules (this was a fundamental finding). This meant that adenine plus guanine was always equal to cytosine and thymine (A + G = C + T). He also found the number of adenine molecules was always equal to the number of thymine molecules (A = T), and the number of guanine molecules was always equal to the number of cytosine molecules (G = C). This became a valuable clue to information found later that would provide the information needed to solve the genetic code.

In 1951, American chemist Linus Carl Pauling worked on protein structures, using X-ray diffraction and his own previous studies of the way in which atoms fit together. He showed that chains of amino acids would twist into the shape of a helix (like the shape of a spiral staircase). This gave another important clue as to how a DNA molecule was shaped, and bio scientists began to seek the final shape of the DNA, keeping this helix in mind. (53)

### The Double Helix

Two scientists who were particularly interested in the possibility of DNA helixes were an Englishman, Francis Harry Crick, and his American coworker, James Dewey Watson. They tried different types of helixes, but none seemed suitable. A helix had to twist according to the natural way in which the atoms fit together. It had to be the kind of helix that would explain the X-ray diffraction images. What they needed were good X-ray diffraction images of pure DNA, but those weren't easy to obtain (52).

As it happened, at the place where Crick and Watson were working there was a New Zealand-born biochemist, Maurice Hugh Frederick Wilkins. He prepared pure DNA fibers that would be expected to produce particularly good X-ray diffraction images. Working for him was English chemist Rosalind Elsie Franklin, who used Wilkins's DNA fibers to make the very best X-ray diffraction images that had yet been taken. Franklin was a very cautious scientist and didn't wish to hurry in figuring out the meaning of her images. She did not want to make any mistakes, nor did she want anyone else to see them while she was thinking out their meaning. She instructed Wilkins not to show her X-ray data to anyone.

Wilkins, however, showed her images to Watson and Crick without asking her permission. They (Watson especially) were much less cautious than Franklin, and the images gave them a remarkable idea almost at once.

Watson and Crick decided that whereas a protein molecule was made up of a chain of amino acids, a DNA molecule was made up of a double chain of nucleotides. This became known as the famous double helix. The two chains of nucleotides were so arranged that the purine and pyrimidine portions faced each other and pointed toward the center of this double chain. This is shown below in figure 4. (Isn't it beautiful?)

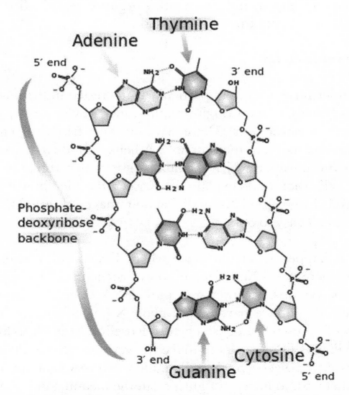

**Figure 4 shows the chemical composition of the helix.**

Notice in this structure that the G to C and A to T are held together by the hydrogen bonds as previously discussed. (51) The hydrogen bond is much weaker than the ordinary bonds that hold atoms together in a molecule. It is strong enough to hold the two nucleotide chains together under ordinary circumstances, but at crucial moments, the two chains can be pulled apart. This is ideal for replication. The two chains are, in fact, like the opposite teeth of a zipper. The zipper usually holds together under the proper conditions, but when you pull down the slide, the two sides of the zipper pull apart easily. This analogy will help you to envision what happens during replication (the function of splitting apart and producing two cells where there was only one).

In order to even the space between the nucleotide chains, a double-ring purine on one side must always be opposite a single-ring pyrimidine. This makes the space between the nucleotide chains just wide enough to hold three rings together at every position. If a purine faced a purine with their two rings each, there wouldn't be enough room, because there would be a total of four rings across and this would be too big. If a pyrimidine faced a pyrimidine, with their single rings each, they wouldn't reach across. Either way, the two chains wouldn't cling together properly at those points. (50) These observations were brought forth by Watson and Crick in their findings.

Hydrogen bonds hold adenine and thymine together quite well, and they also hold together guanine and cytosine. On one nucleotide chain, the order can be anything, but on the other side, there must always be a matching (complementary) set of purines or pyrimidines: C for G, T for A, and vice versa. If the arrangement on one nucleotide is A, G, A, T, T, C, G, G, G, C, then on the other it must be T, C, T, A, A, G, C, C, C, G. It's as simple as that—just match the complement of the arrangement seen on one side (just like the zipper mentioned). As we discuss how these codes are passed, you will understand how these complements work.

This explains why Chargaff (previously discussed) had found that in DNA molecules there were always equal numbers of adenines and thymines and equal number of guanines and cytosines.

Finally, the two chains were twisted in such a way as to produce a double helix. They were like two spiral staircases, twisting together, with the banister of one just fitting between the curves of the other. See figure 6 below.

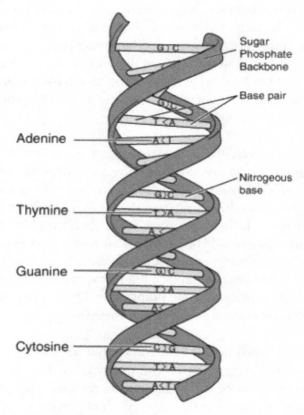

Base pairs, of a DNA double helix

Figure 5. Double helix, showing A to T and G to C pairs and showing the base pairs of adenine, thymine, guanine, and cytosine between the two "banisters."

The backbone of the DNA strand is made from alternating phosphate and sugar residues. (62) The sugar in DNA is 2-deoxyribose, which is a pentose (five carbons) sugar. The sugars are joined together by phosphate groups that form *phosphodiester bonds* between the third and fifth carbon atoms of adjacent sugar rings. These asymmetric bonds mean a strand of DNA has a direction. In a double helix, the direction of the nucleotides in one strand is opposite that in the other nucleotide strand. This arrangement of DNA strands is called antiparallel. The asymmetric ends of DNA strands are referred to as the 5' (five prime) and 3' (three prime) ends. (23) Two of the major differences between DNA and RNA are the sugar previously mentioned and uracil in place of thymine. Also review figure 4; of course, RNA is not in a double helix but is a single strand.

Watson and Crick described this double helix structure of DNA in 1953, and it made a sensation at once. (62) Watson, Crick, and Wilkins all shared the Nobel Prize for medicine and physiology in 1962. Franklin might have been honored too, but she had died four years earlier, and the Nobel Prize is never presented posthumously.

Watson and Crick not only described the double helix structure, they also worked out many of the features of this double helix and how the base pairs worked. They described the directions of the backbones and the antiparallel structure of the backbones of the structure.

The structure worked out by Watson and Crick explained how DNA molecules produced replicas of themselves when cells divided. Because each DNA molecule can produce another just like itself, skin cells can divide into two skin cells, liver cells can divide into two liver cells, and so on. It's why egg cells have DNA molecules like those of the mother, sperm cells like those of the father, and resulting young have DNA molecules and characteristics like those of both parents.

### *Replication—Cell Division*

Here's how it works. When a cell is ready to divide, the two chains of the double helix begin to pull apart at the hydrogen bonds. This is made easy, as mentioned earlier, due to the hydrogen bonds, which are fairly weak. (51) Here are figures 3 and 4 again so you can see the bonds.

At top, a **GC** base pair with three hydrogen bonds. At the bottom, **AT** base pair with two hydrogen bonds. Hydrogen bonds are shown as dashed lines.

As hydrogen bonds are not covalent (covalent bonding is when two atoms share one or more of their valence electrons. The valence electrons are the ones in the outermost shell of the atom. This forms a strong bond.), they can be broken and rejoined. The helix can therefore be pulled apart like a zipper; complementarity, all the information in the double-stranded sequence of a DNA helix, is duplicated on each strand, which is vital in DNA replication. Indeed, this reversible and specific interaction between complementary base pairs is critical for all the functions of DNA in living organisms.[1]

The two types of base pairs form different numbers of hydrogen bonds, AT forming two hydrogen bonds, and GC forming three hydrogen bonds (see figures). The GC base pair is therefore stronger than the AT base pair. As a result, it is both the percentage of GC base pairs and the overall length of a DNA double helix that determine the strength of the association between the two strands of DNA. Long DNA helices with a high GC content have stronger-interacting strands, while short helices with high AT content have weaker-interacting strands. Parts of the DNA double helix that need to separate easily, such as the TATAAT Pribnow box in bacterial promoters, tend to have sequences with a high AT content, making the strands easier to pull apart. In the laboratory, the strength of this interaction can be measured by finding the temperature required to break the hydrogen bonds, their melting temperature (also called $T_m$ value). (89) When all the base pairs in a DNA double helix melt, the strands separate and exist in solution as two entirely independent molecules. These single-stranded DNA molecules have no single common shape, but some conformations are more stable than others.]

Look at figure 4 above. The hydrogen bonds are shown between the purines and the pyrimidines, and you can see where it is easily detached, one side from the complementary side. The nucleotides along each chain quickly pick up single nucleotides that are present in the cell fluids (the fluid is made up of many purines and pyrimidines) of the nucleus. It picks up its complement, as previously discussed, so as to maintain not only the integrity of the code, but also the spacing between the backbones of the double helix that are made up of the sugar molecules. It is important that this spacing remains constant as well. When a guanine-cytosine base pair pulls apart, the guanine picks up a new cytosine from the nucleotides in the nucleus fluid almost immediately; the same action occurs when an adenine-thymine base pair pulls apart. They therefore complete the replication. This occurs throughout the whole DNA structure as the chromosomes split and form two identical chromosomes. In this way two complete chromosomes result, and after the pulling apart and splitting, the DNA within each is identical. Keep in mind that this occurs in all the cells of the body. This is a miraculous undertaking.

The other unique feature of this double helix structure is that it can fold like an accordion into a short pile in the small nucleus of each chromosome, taking up very little room while achieving the tasks it is to perform. The DNA chain is 22 to 26 Angstroms wide (2.2 to 2.6 nanometers—billionths of an inch), and one nucleotide unit is 3.3 Angstroms (0.33 nanometers) long. Although each individual repeating unit is very small, DNA polymers can be enormous molecules containing millions of nucleotides. For instance, the largest, chromosome number 1, is 220 million base pairs long. Think of a chain as a long word. Remember, the DNA is responsible for the entire genetic code. This means it has to be able to "write" many words, all of different lengths. Each of these words will mean something relative to what the DNA wants to happen in the body. These words represent instructions to produce certain amino acids and compose certain proteins. Keep in mind that all the cells of your body are physically alike and the entire nucleus and their DNA are alike. This means the cells in your heart are the same as the cells in your muscles. However, they have to perform quite differently. It's amazing to me that after conception these cells must make all the parts of the human body and somehow know which ones will be heart cells and which are going to be muscle cells.

The nucleotide repeats (in the double helix the same base can be repeated, such as CA, CA, CA tied to the backbone and to its complement on the complementary side of the double helix) contain both the segment of the backbone of the molecule, which holds the chain together, and a base, which interacts with the other DNA strand in the helix, its complementary nucleotide. In general, a base linked to a sugar is called a *nucleoside,* and a base linked to both a sugar and one or more phosphate groups is called a *nucleotide.* If multiple nucleotides are linked together, as in DNA, this polymer is referred to as a *polynucleotide.* The backbone of the DNA strand is made from alternating phosphate and sugar residues. The sugar in DNA is 2-deoxyribose, which is a carbon sugar. The sugars are joined together by phosphate groups that form phosphodiester bonds between the third and fifth carbon atoms of adjacent sugar rings. These asymmetric bonds mean a strand of DNA has a direction. In a double helix, the direction of the nucleotides in one strand is opposite to their direction in the other strand. As previously indicate the arrangement of DNA strands is called antiparallel.

Although scientists recognized the structure of the DNA as distinct from RNA, it was unclear how it worked and how it related to the genetic code. It was understood how this busy nucleus caused certain proteins to be formed. So the question became; "What's the code, and how does it work?"

We have covered how replications occur and affect all the chromosomes in the body, but we haven't discovered how DNA controls the generation of amino acids and the structuring of the proteins in the body—the sought-after secret.

The order of the nucleotides that we just reviewed is different for every human being. It is so representative of an individual that we now use it like fingerprints; we now use DNA to solve mysteries. It is better than fingerprints, but how does it work? Bio scientists wanted to solve that also. The order of the nucleotides, with their G's and T's and A's and C's, must be the key. This key must control the order of the amino acids required to provide the proteins needed by the human body.

There are four different nucleotides (adenine, guanine, thymine, and cytosine). Can they determine the information to select the amino acids? There are twenty-two amino acids, and we have four nucleotides. In order to solve this problem, think about today's personal computers ... or all computers, for that matter. They work using just ones and zeros. However, these ones and zeros can do much more than the twenty-six letters of the alphabet. It's just a matter of how the ones and zeros are generated and sequenced. With one sequence they mean one thing, and with another sequence they mean something quite different.

But maybe more important than the number of nucleotides and their codes is how they get out of the nucleus of the chromosomes. The nucleus of the human chromosome has DNA inside, and the nucleus shell that surrounds this core of DNA is impervious to DNA passing through it. But remember that I told you that the chromosome of the eukaryotes (humans, animals, plants) has an outer membrane that we can call one enclosure; between it and the shell that surrounds the nucleus are other structures that I told you I would discuss later. Well, this is later. I'll discuss what's in between these two walls. However, I won't go into it in too detailed a manner, or it would take up another book. So I will cover the basics.

In 1956, Romanian-American biochemist George Emil Palade found the place where the enzymes are located. Using an electron microscope, a tool that could magnify structures about a thousand times more than a conventional microscope, he found tiny structures within the cytoplasm, the sea of material between the outer membrane of a cell and the nucleus shell, in which many small structures are located. There are upwards of 150,000 of them in every cell, and this is where the enzymes are produced. He found each of these structures also contained RNA, and he called these structures ribosomes. Palade received the Nobel Prize for physiology and medicine in 1974. (50)

To learn about the ribosomes and their locations within a cell, review the diagram below in figure 6. (63)

**Eukaryotic Cells**

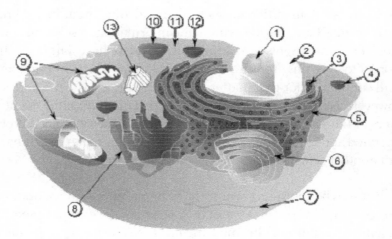

Figure 6 Diagram of a typical eukaryotic cell,
showing subcellular components. Organelles: (1) nucleolus;
(2) nucleus; (3) ribosome; (4) vesicle; (5) rough endoplasmic
reticulum (ER); (6) Golgi apparatus; (7) cytoskeleton; (8)
smooth ER; (9) mitochondria; (10) vacuole; (11) cytoplasm;
(12) lysosome; (13) centrioles within centrosome. (63)

The diagram of a typical eukaryotic cell (figure 6 above) shows what would be found in animals, humans, and plants—all have a similar cell. The key difference between the eukaryotic cell and the prokaryotic cells found in bacteria and viruses is that the eukaryote cell has a nucleus. It's within this nucleus that the chromosomes and DNA are located. There are twenty-three chromosome pairs within the nucleus. The parts diagrammed in figure 6 that we are interested in now are the (1) nucleolus, (2) nucleus, (3) ribosome, and (11) cytoplasm. These relate to where the DNA is located in the nucleus. The RNA is located within the ribosome, with some in the nucleus. The cytoplasm is the material between the outer membrane of the cell and the nucleus shell. Cytoplasm contains the various other organelles, comparable to organs in our bodies like the heart, lungs, etc. Organelles, likewise, perform organlike functions in the cytoplasm. To discuss them fully is beyond the scope of this book.

If you want to learn more about the functions of the various sections of the eukaryotic cell, visit the following Web site: (http://en.wikipedia.org/wiki/Cell_Biology), where a complete description is given.

Palade's work provided information about the ribosomes, without answering how the information gets from the DNA to these ribosomes. Palade's findings, along with information determined by Watson and Crick and the Russian-American scientist George Gamow (who I personally believe was a genius in many areas of science), began to reveal the answer. Gamow suggested that it was not the individual G, A, T, or C that determined the code, but a group of them. He used great logic in reviewing this. He claimed that if you used only these four, the most codes DNA could offer would be sixteen. Any two of the four nucleotides such as TA, GA, etc., would only create sixteen combinations. He knew that sixteen was not enough to decode to produce twenty-two amino acids. He suggested that three nucleotides at a time would create sixty-four combinations that could then be decoded to provide more than enough to produce the enzymes and twenty-two amino acids. So his solution was triplets, and that's how the genetic code must be passed from the DNA in the nucleus. What Palade showed in 1956 was not only where the enzymes were located, but also where significant amounts of RNA were located.

# The Way into the Nucleus

In 1961, two French biochemists, Jacques Lucien Monod and Francois Jacob, suggested that RNA was the answer to that question. After all, RNA is found both in the nucleus and in the cytoplasm, and in the ribosomes in particular. (53) RNA has a structure just like DNA, except that it has ribose instead of deoxyribose and uracil instead of thymine. When a DNA molecule replicates, it might, every once in a while, form an RNA nucleotide chain, instead of another DNA nucleotide chain. The RNA nucleotide chain would have its nucleotides in the exact order of the DNA nucleotide chain except that uracil (U) would be found where thymine (T) had been. Since the RNA is not a double helix, it must take the nucleotides off the DNA in a series. But how would a single strand of nucleotides representing the double helix with the nucleotide pairs perform this? This would be reviewed and answered. The molecule of RNA would slip out of the nucleus and would serve as the messenger, carrying the DNA information to the ribosomes. This molecule of RNA came to be known as *messenger RNA* (mRNA).

It is important to remember the other things about RNA that are different from DNA. The RNA is not in a double helix formation but in a linear one. Whereas the DNA has two base pairs between the two backbones of the DNA, the RNA is not limited. It is a linear molecule and therefore can continuously take the base pairs and line them up on the ribose sugar backbone in single-file order. (Later it was determined that it would take half pairs from one of the backbone strands for the RNA messenger.) As an example, if ten base pairs were to be taken off the DNA, they would be shown in order one after the other as ten nucleotides in series on the RNA ribose single backbone. This is very important; remember that Gamow had said that the code had to come off as triplets. This is not possible with DNA, where only pairs come off. The series of nucleotides on the RNA could be taken off in triplets; it's just a matter of nature providing a method of cutting these single strands every third nucleotide.

Another major difference is that the RNA can pass through the nucleus shell and the DNA cannot. The DNA stays within the nucleus shell to protect it from changing. It's possible the DNA with its double backbones cannot pass through the semipermeable shell because it has a broader and more complex structure than the single-backbone RNA; perhaps the fluid of the deoxyribonucleic acid is blocked whereas the ribonucleic acid is not. There is also a difference of one nucleotide, where uracil (U) replaces thymine (T). However, it turns out that this is not what is intended by Mother Nature, and you will soon see why. It is important for the DNA to stay in the nucleus and not to change. It is the key to one's life from the very beginning when one is formed during the sex act.

Both Monod and Jacob received the 1965 Nobel Prize for medicine and physiology. Prior to Monod and Jacob's work, Spanish-American biochemist Severo Ochoa had discovered an enzyme that acted to tie nucleotides together to form an RNA chain. This made it possible to make synthetic RNA. Ochoa received a share of the 1959 Nobel Prize for medicine and physiology. This played a part in the progression of successes in solving the riddle of the DNA/RNA issue. Using the information that Ochoa, Monod, and Jacob had developed concerning the messenger RNA, American biochemist Marshall Warren Nirenberg manufactured synthetic messenger RNA. By choosing which nucleotides to start with, he could make messenger RNA with particular triplets. He would then find out which particular amino acids would be produced in a nucleotide chain by these triplets. He knew if he could convert these triplets into an amino acid, then he could determine which amino acid it represented and eventually the protein it produced. This was all done by known chemicals in test tubes. In this way, Nirenberg began to break the genetic code. He started with a polyuridic acid and added it to several systems containing other known enzymes and ribosomes. Eventually out of one of the mixtures came a known protein. By carefully choosing several known nucleotides, he arrived at all the amino acids and their related proteins. He discovered which nucleotide triplet, called a codon, produced which amino acid. By 1967, every nucleotide codon was tied to a particular amino acid, and the genetic code was completely worked out, although the method of it still was not complete. (53) Nirenberg and Indian-American chemist Har Gobind Khorana received shares of the 1968 Nobel Prize for medicine and physiology.

While Nirenberg was working on the genetic code, another American biochemist, Mahlon Bush Hoagland, was locating small RNA molecules in the cytoplasm (material between the nucleus wall and the outer membrane of the cell). (53) These were double-ended molecules. At one end was a nucleotide triplet (anticodon) that would fit a particular codon on the messenger RNA (like a zipper, as I previously mentioned). On the other end was a portion that attached itself to a particular amino acid located in the cytoplasm. Because they transferred the information from the anticodon triplet to the amino acid, such molecules are called *transfer RNA* (tRNA).

Putting these pieces of information together, bio scientists could determine the complete function. It is the sequence of these four bases along the backbone that encodes information in the form of codons on the messenger RNA. This information is read using the genetic code, which specifies the sequence of the amino acids within proteins. The code of the DNA is read by copying stretches of DNA into the related nucleic acid RNA, in a process called *transcription*. Transcription forms the messenger RNA (mRNA). Compare this to writing words. You take the letters of the alphabet and you combine them into words. The process of transcription is the same within the cell. The codons are like the letters of the alphabet. A combination of codons forms a word coming from the nucleus. This is the message emanating from the nucleus via the messenger RNA.

### *Transcription and mRNA*

RNA polymerase (an enzyme) opens the part of the DNA to be transcribed. This is like the action of unzipping a zipper. This RNA polymerase acts to unzip the double strand into single strands. Keep in mind that the base pairs are held by the double backbone of the double helix. These backbones are called the strands. (54) There are two of them with the information between them in the pairs we discussed. By unzipping, the two backbones are split from a double helix to single strands, with each strand having one backbone and combined with half a pair forming one-half of the information in the strand. This can be seen in figure 7 below. Remember, the backbone (strands) move in opposite directions, so the top backbone comes off as the mRNA as shown in figure 7.

Notice when the triplet comes off as ATG it is now coming out as AUG, since there is no T outside the nucleus and it is replaced by the U as we discussed, as uracil.

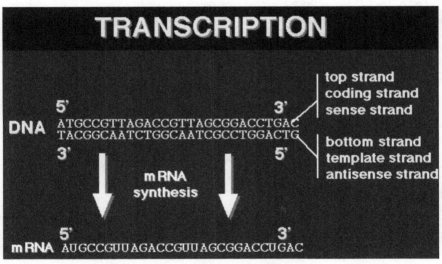

Figure 7 shows the double-strand DNA going off as a single strand on the messenger RNA (mRNA).

As mentioned, the code consists of at least three bases, according to astronomer George Gamow. To code for the twenty essential amino acids, a genetic code must consist of at least a three-base set (triplet) of the four bases. If one considers the possibilities of arranging four things, three at a time (4x4x4), there are sixty-four possible code words, or codons (a three-base sequence on the mRNA that codes for either a specific amino acid or a control word). With the mRNA coming off in a serial fashion, it can form codons, such as AUG or CCG, for example.

One strand of the double-stranded DNA is called the *bottom strand*, or *template strand*, or *antisense* strand, as shown in figure 7. This strand is tied to one-half of the base pairs, or codons that are transcribed into the messenger RNA (mRNA). The other strand is called the *top strand, coding strand*, or *sense strand*, as shown in figure 7. This contains the other half pairs called the anticodons, which become the transfer RNA (tRNA). The anticodons are therefore the complements of the codons, just as they were when they were together as base pairs in the double helix. Only one strand of DNA (template strand) is transcribed as shown in figure 7 and comes off as the mRNA (messenger RNA). RNA nucleotides are available in the region of the chromatin (this process only occurs during interphase) and are linked together similarly to the DNA process.

As can be seen in figure 7, the codons are no longer associated as base pairs but become a string of mRNA. This allows them to be decoded in triplets as mRNA.

Likewise, the transfer anticodons are no longer associated as base pairs but become a string of anticodons that were taken from the opposite strand of the DNA that the mRNA took; so it's the complement. Like the mRNA, the tRNA anticodons can move through the nucleus shell and do so in another direction. Each of these streams of codons and anticodons move through the nucleus shell at different points.

These are done in series on the messenger RNA shown in figure 8. (54) Note that wherever there is a T on the coding strand (top strand), there will be a U on the mRNA strand. (Refer to figure 8 again, since recognizing the U in place of the T makes it easier to see what is happening.) This is because the RNA does not have thymine but has uracil in its place, as discussed previously. The messenger RNA is transcribed as indicated with the copy of a section of the

DNA molecule. The mRNA travels through the nucleus shell to the ribosome, where tRNA has transferred amino molecules that attach themselves at the various anticodons of the messenger RNA. The anticodons formed in the transfer RNA were from the coding strand and are the complements of the template strand and therefore form a perfect mate.

To summarize the cycle that occurs: the DNA contains the code. The code is unzipped into two strands. The messenger RNA (mRNA) reads the code and therefore contains the blueprint for construction of a protein. The complement other half of the unzipped code, tRNA, is transferred out of the nucleus. The mRNA moves through the nucleus shell to the ribosome. The ribosomal (rRNA) is the construction site where the protein is made, and transfer RNA (tRNA) is the truck delivering the proper amino acid to the site at the right time. From this a protein is generated. The mRNA and the tRNA are the complementary halves of the DNA and make their way out of the nucleus with their information for manufacturing the amino acids which eventually produce the proteins.

Transfer RNAs (anticodons) were studied carefully by American chemist Robert William Holley. He purified several varieties in 1962. By 1965, he actually put the proper nucleotide together and synthesized one of them. In 1968, he shared the Nobel Prize with Nirenberg and Khorana. Nirenberg's group was able to determine the sequences of fifty-four out of sixty-four codons. Subsequent work by Har Gobind Khorana identified the rest of the code, and Holley determined the structure of transfer RNA, the adapter molecule that facilitates translation.(53) Each anticodon gets the transfer RNA molecule that happens to fit that particular codon and no other. Amino acids attach to the other end of each transfer RNA, but only the amino acid that specifically fits that end of that particular transfer RNA. The amino acids then all hook together to create a particular protein molecule. The DNA has done its duty of sending a message via the mRNA and the complementary transfer tRNA to complement the mRNA and pick up the proper amino acids called out by the DNA.

You can now envision the DNA in its shell passing out instructions one after the other, determined by the genetic code that is held within its genes. This is amazing enough, but you have to remember that DNA was present at the conception of the new baby. It handles the building of the baby from time zero until the time of death. It even has encoded within its genes when that child will go into puberty and eventually become a grown man or woman. Isn't this a wonder?

# The Genetic Code: Translation of RNA Code into Protein

The genetic code was broken by Marshall Nirenberg and Heinrich Matthaeus a decade after Watson and Crick's work (1953). Nirenberg discovered that RNA, regardless of its source organism, could initiate protein synthesis when combined with contents of broken *Escherichia. coli* cells. (54) By adding poly-U to each of twenty test tubes (each tube having a different "tagged" amino acid), Nirenberg and Matthaeus were able to determine that the codon UUU (the only one in poly-U) coded for the amino acid phenylalanine (see figure 8).

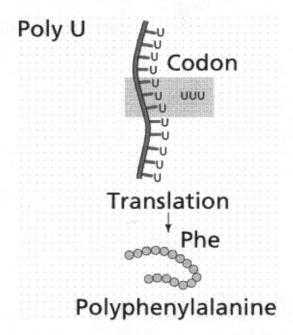

Figure 8. Steps in breaking the genetic code:
the deciphering of a poly-U mRNA.

Image (90)

Likewise, an artificial mRNA consisting of alternating A and C bases would code for alternating amino acids histidine and threonine (figure 10). Gradually, a complete listing of the genetic code codons was developed. (54)

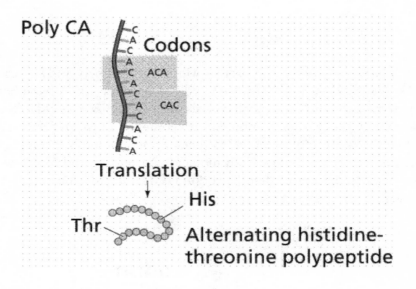

Figure 9. Deciphering the code: poly CAC to histidine-threonine polypeptide. (90)

The genetic code consists of sixty-one amino-acid coding codons and three termination codons, which stop the process of translation. The genetic code is thus redundant (degenerate in the sense of having multiple states amounting to the same thing), with, for example, glycine coded for by GGU, GGC, GGA, and GGG codons. If a codon is mutated, say from GGU to CGU, is the same amino acid specified?

The genetic code has redundancy but no ambiguity. (57) For example, although codon GAA and GAG both specify glutamic acid (redundancy), neither of them specifies any other amino acid (no ambiguity). Only two amino acids are specified by a single codon; one of these is the amino acid methionine, specified by the codon AUG, which also specifies the start of translation; the other is tryptophan, specified by the codon UGG. The degeneracy of the genetic code is what accounts for the existence of silent mutations.

Review the complete code of sixty-four codons shown below in figure 10. Inside the squares is marked the amino acid that will be picked up by the code. This is how twenty-two amino acids are picked that will then be used to generate the proteins. Note on the left side is the letter that will appear as the first letter of the triplet code (codon). The second letter is determined by the horizontal U, C, A, G at the top of the chart. The third letter of the codon is determined by the letters going down the right side of the chart; amino acids formed by each code are shown. (54)

## Second letter

| | | U | | C | | A | | G | | |
|---|---|---|---|---|---|---|---|---|---|---|
| **First letter** | **U** | UUU UUC | Phenyl-alanine | UCU UCC | Serine | UAU UAC | Tyrosine | UGU UGC | Cysteine | U C |
| | | UUA UUG | Leucine | UCA UCG | | UAA UAG | Stop codon Stop codon | UGA UGG | Stop codon Tryptophan | A G |
| | **C** | CUU CUC CUA CUG | Leucine | CCU CCC CCA CCG | Proline | CAU CAC | Histidine | CGU CGC CGA CGG | Arginine | U C A G |
| | | | | | | CAA CAG | Glutamine | | | |
| | **A** | AUU AUC AUA | Isoleucine | ACU ACC ACA | Threonine | AAU AAC | Asparagine | AGU AGC | Serine | U C |
| | | AUG | Methionine; initiation codon | ACG | | AAA AAG | Lysine | AGA AGG | Arginine | A G |
| | **G** | GUU GUC GUA GUG | Valine | GCU GCC GCA GCG | Alanine | GAU GAC | Aspartic acid | GGU GGC GGA GGG | Glycine | U C A G |
| | | | | | | GAA GAG | Glutamic acid | | | |

Third **Letter**

Figure 10. The genetic code. (91)

tRNA carries the proper amino acid to the ribosome when the codons call for them. There are sixty-one different tRNAs, each having a different binding site for the amino acid and a different anticodon. For the codon UUU, the complementary anticodon is

AAA. Energy for binding the amino acid to tRNA comes from ATP's conversion (adenosine triphosphate, which we discussed early in the book as the universal energy element in the human body) to adenosine monophosphate (AMP).

The illustration below (figure 11) is from Genentech's Access Excellence site. The drawing is available at http://www.gene.com/ ae/AB/GG/protein_synthesis.html

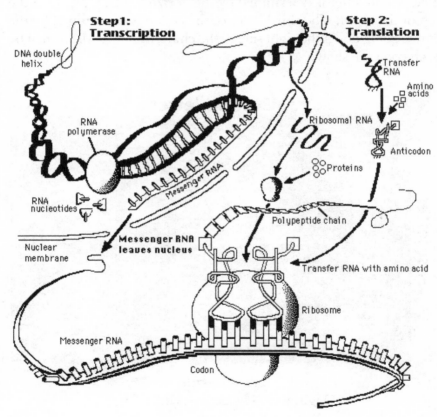

Figure 11. Protein synthesis
http://www.estrellamountain.edu/faculty/
farabee/biobk/protein_synthesis.gif
This diagram shows how proteins are synthesized. (54)

Start from the upper left part of the schematic. Step 1 is the transcription, which is activated by the RNA polymerase. The messenger RNA transcribes the DNA by taking one-half of the pairs from the backbone of the double helix. Notice, as mentioned, that the mRNA only takes half pairs of the nucleotides and, as codons, transports them in series rather than the complementary pair in the double helix. While the mRNA proceeds through the nuclear shell on the one path that carries the codons to the ribosome, Step 2 shows the tRNA (upper right-hand corner of the schematic) and its anticodons passing through the nuclear membrane, picking up the amino acids and taking them to the ribosome to meet with its particular codon. The ribosomal RNA passes through the nuclear membrane and arrives at the ribosome, where the proteins are manufactured. (28).

## Number of Genes in the Human

Human cells have twenty-three pairs of large linear nuclear chromosomes, for a total of forty-six per cell. Sequencing the human genome over the past few years has provided a great deal of information about the number of genes in each of the of the chromosome pairs. Below is a table (figure 13) compiling statistics for the number of genes, the total bases, and the sequenced bases. (55)

| Chromosome | Genes | Total bases | Sequenced bases |
|---|---|---|---|
| 1 | 3,148 | 247,200,000 | 224,999,719 |
| 2 | 902 | 242,750,000 | 237,712,649 |
| 3 | 1,436 | 199,450,000 | 194,704,827 |
| 4 | 453 | 191,260,000 | 187,297,063 |
| 5 | 609 | 180,840,000 | 177,702,766 |
| 6 | 1,585 | 170,900,000 | 167,273,992 |
| 7 | 1,824 | 158,820,000 | 154,952,424 |
| 8 | 781 | 146,270,000 | 142,612,826 |
| 9 | 1,229 | 140,440,000 | 120,312,298 |
| 10 | 1,312 | 135,370,000 | 131,624,737 |
| 11 | 405 | 134,450,000 | 131,130,853 |
| 12 | 1,330 | 132,290,000 | 130,303,534 |
| 13 | 623 | 114,130,000 | 95,559,980 |

| 14 | 886 | 106,360,000 | 88,290,585 |
| 15 | 676 | 100,340,000 | 81,341,915 |
| 16 | 898 | 88,820,000 | 78,884,754 |
| 17 | 1,367 | 78,650,000 | 77,800,220 |
| 18 | 365 | 76,120,000 | 74,656,155 |
| 19 | 1,553 | 63,810,000 | 55,785,651 |
| 20 | 816 | 62,440,000 | 59,505,254 |
| 21 | 446 | 46,940,000 | 34,171,998 |
| 22 | 595 | 49,530,000 | 34,893,953 |
| X (sex chromosome) | 1,093 | 154,910,000 | 151,058,754 |
| Y (sex chromosome) | 125 | 57,740,000 | 22,429,293 |

Figure 12. Chromosomes and number of genes per chromosome
http://en.wikipedia.org/wiki/Chromosome.

Keep in mind that there are twenty-two amino acids, but there are an infinite number of proteins that can be made from the combinations of the amino acids. The table above shows how the codons provide the twenty-two amino acids. The sequencing of the different amino acids determines the actions that take place to generate the proteins. The amino acids are like words, and the proteins are like sentences. There is a complete paragraph that determines how the various proteins are generated and sent to do their service in the body.

I am an electrical engineer by education. This method that the chromosome's DNA uses to send out codons via the mRNA to provide given actions is quite similar to how a microprocessor works. The microprocessor has a CPU in its center, which is like the DNA inside the nucleus. The CPU—central processing unit—can add, subtract, multiply, divide, and do logic. However, it needs an operating program to tell it how to do the functions it does. This is done by programming ROM (read-only memory) codes that provide the operating program for the CPU. These ROM codes are built into the microprocessor and do not change. In that respect they are like the DNA that one is provided at birth and doesn't change. We will learn later that the DNA can be changed by a retrovirus, but this is a disease. Likewise, a ROM code in a computer is not supposed to change, but accidents happen to it like they do to the DNA. The ROM code provides the program for the CPU to do the various functions as it receives information from the input to the microprocessor. This program of the operating system is like the genetic code of a human. It will only do what it has been coded to do. The program is a sequencer of sorts. It tells how to handle various sequences. Meanwhile, while the functions are being carried out, the CPU sends messages to the memory and recalls messages back from the memory, depending on the function that has been programmed. The CPU makes decisions based on what has been programmed into it, relating to the information (data) coming in.

In a living cell, the genetic code is the code that is built in and won't change (unless a mutation occurs). It is similar to the program built into the microprocessor. It sequences through the various codons via the mRNA and completes the buildup via the tRNA of the proteins. However, it doesn't keep putting out the same information all the time. The body is a dynamic system, and it may need changes, depending on the stresses placed on it. These stresses depend on which of the millions of alleles (code addresses, which are sort of like the random access memory [RAM] of the microprocessor) are called upon for a response. The alleles are the like the addresses within each chromosome. See table 2 above, which shows the number of genes in each chromosome.

### Conclusion on Cells and DNA/RNA

I tried to achieve the difficult task of describing the way the chromosomes, genes, and genetic code work as simply as possible for the layman to understand. I am not a bio scientist, so in that respect I am a layman, and I presented it as I understand it. I am a retired professional electrical engineer who was involved in the development of integrated circuits over forty-five years (1959–2002), including the solid state physics involved, and I understand technical information. From this background, after much research, I have tried to supply the reader with my interpretation of the events. I find it truly amazing that a difficult problem that took so many years for scientists to track down could be tied together in a manner that is fairly easy to understand. Isn't that the way of life? That is, when something as complicated as this is established, it looks easy when one looks backward in time. This was probably the toughest puzzle for the bio scientists and chemists to put together, yet once they got the basics done, it is presented in fairly simple form. I added the names and the countries of the people that made significant contributions toward this complex picture; they look like a football team that was working together for one purpose, and they came up with it. Of course the details I left out of this book are too complex to try to cover in this book, so I provided enough to give an understanding of the process. It would take another book to go into the details.

# The Human Genome

Even when scientists reached this level of understanding in determining the genome of man, it took many years and computer hours to put that whole genetic code (genome) together. There was a federal government program to decipher the code, and a separate private concern headed up by Craig Venter, head of Celera, both racing to beat each other. (56) It didn't start out that way. It started with the government program, and then the private concern worked to do it faster with their approach. I believe in the end that each helped the other. It was about a fifteen-year venture to reach as far as I have discussed. The completion of the human genome led to mapping other genomes to see how they compared with that of humans. They tackled the mouse and found it had almost the same genome as man. Isn't that something?

As complex as the cell is, with its DNA and RNA and the resultant amino acids and the building of proteins, it's even more complex when one considers that every cell in the human body is exactly the same, yet none carry out functions the same way. For example, a cell in the skin is the same as a cell in the brain and a cell in the arm muscle, yet the neurons in the brain do not act like the arm muscle or the skin tissue. Here is a key secret. Although the cells are the same throughout the body, they are controlled by some kind of switches in their location that make them work the way they do for that location. It's like the cells in the muscles see different switches for turning on special sections of the chromosomes and only use those to perform their functions. In that respect it's comparable, as I mentioned earlier, to the microprocessor, which functions so similarly to the workings of the nucleus and the various parts of the cell to perform a task. Microprocessors are used for many tasks. It's a matter in many cases of how the human addresses the microprocessor as to how it performs a given function. If the operator wants one thing, he provides data to certain portions of the processor. If he wants it to be used different **severe acute respiratory syndrome**, he puts a different code into the same processor, and it performs that task, most of the time only requiring one different button to be chosen for a completely different function. Likewise, each cell in its physical position performs a completely different function than if it were in some other place in the body. But it isn't anywhere else—it's wherever it is, and the thing that changes is the code or human function switch at that location.

We know that, although identical at every location, the cell controls the amino acids and the construction of proteins that are probably different for each physical location of the cell. For example, the cells in the brain do not have to do the functions that the muscle in the arm does, so different amino acids and proteins are generated in the brain. The question that I have as a layman is, What is it that allows the cell to identify its location and what is required of the cells at that location?

In the beginning, when an embryo is just a set of chromosomes made up of the male and female contributions, it begins to replicate while in the mother's body. As this replication expands and cells are formed, the embryo grows. From the embryo to the formation of a complete child, it is a wonder that each of these replications becomes a different part of the body and begins to function as individual parts of the body while taking food from the mother. This continues while the baby is in the mother's body and after birth. However, after birth, there are no new things that grow; the ones already there begin to take on growth. Somehow, the body knows that it doesn't have to add any more new things, just take in nutrition and let the body grow.

Males and females both go through puberty, bringing changes to their bodies and their lives. Sex organs change, and both voices change, the male's more than the female's. His voice transforms to a deeper tone; this is another thing that differentiates the male from the female. This transformation within the male and female is the first step in becoming an adult and makes it possible to start another human being—which more or less begins the sequence all over again. The male and female through sex can produce another human being, but it will be different than either of the two in some ways.

Prior to reaching this stage, neither males nor females are able to reproduce. The male has no sperm to generate, and although the female has eggs, they are not released until puberty is reached. Then each month the female body releases an egg. If it is not fertilized, it leaves the female in the form of blood. This is sometimes called "the disappointment of the uterus." But eventually most females have their egg fertilized by male sperm, and the chromosome combination becomes the start of a new life.

This reaching of maturity or adulthood reminds me of the Mendel experiments with self-pollinating pea plants. They eventually flower and produce pollen, which contains the male gametes, which fall on the female parts of the plant, which are not yet prepared to accept this sperm. But the pollen grain grows a pollen tube, which allows the sperm to travel through the stigma and style to reach the pea plant's ovary. The ripened ovary wall becomes the fruit, or pea pod, of a new plant. In this case the pea plant is self-pollinating and the female has nothing to say about when it is ready; whereas with humans, the male and female have to consent to mate (most of the time) to carry on their expansion of the human race. Whether with a pea plant or a human being, the change is dramatic. How those genomes know what to do after that is amazing.

Back to the discussion about the human genome and what that will bring to mankind. The completed genome, accomplished by either Craig Venter and/or the government program, gave many bioscientists a look into many possibilities. They believed that this insight should show what causes various diseases and what results in different functions between genes in the body. One good thing— they found the genome was smaller than expected. It originally was believed that the human genome was on the order of 150,000 to 200,000 genes. It was found that there are actually 30,000 to 45,000 genes, which can make the problem easier to solve.

Every person is made up of three billion chemical combinations. It took thirteen years and cost about $450 million to finish the first-ever complete detailing of the human genome, in 2003, using a fleet of genetic analysis equipment. Progress got the detailing to only weeks at a cost of about $5 million, mainly due to the existence of this base. I believe it was down to half a million dollars in 2007. Today (2015) a human genome can be completed in a day due to advanced computer programs at a much lower cost. This method is now being used to try to track medical problems where the answer is not available otherwise.

It was found that several mutations can occur; resulting in certain diseases, but to date there has been no progress on finding out how to prevent the diseases. I am sure this will be resolved the more we work on it. Many of these things are found by inputting data into a computer as we find new things, and eventually a program will be written to tie things together. Sometimes this is done by trial and effect. This is much easier with a computer than if done by human effort.

By helping chart the entire human genome, machines for the first time have provided a clear view of the three billion chemical combinations—the nucleotide base pairs we discussed—that make up a human. And since the mapping of the human genome, the power of DNA analysis equipment has steadily increased, making it easier to answer age-old questions about who we are and where we come from—and hopefully how to live longer. Comparisons are being done by the National Geographic Society to trace human migratory routes over the past 150,000 years, and they show how closely related we are, like a big family. The current technology helps us to look backward in time and allows us to determine the evolution of life.

The resolving of the human genome has shown that there are times when more than one gene is responsible for an action. They are somewhat related. We should have realized this, since we found early in the hunt for the genetic code that there is one protein that results in the generation of insulin and another from the same protein that results in the female's organs being better moisturized to allow for easier function during certain female functions. We have to keep in mind that the genome is made up of contributions from both the male and female during conception. Therefore the resulting chromosomes and their genes aren't always those that are just from the male or the female. This being a fact, there are probably times when part of the genome is not used by the male and likewise for the female. I guess that is why for certain diseases one takes several types of medicines that affect different parts of the body in different people.

As I mentioned earlier I have suffered from a dramatic case of very high blood pressure since I was eighteen. In 1966 I was told that if I didn't take care of the problem that I had five years to live. This was due to having a very high reading on the systolic and diastolic readings. What was done to lower the systolic didn't lower the diastolic, and the difference between these two is the pulse pressure. Lowering the high reading without changing the low reading resulted in a drop in pulse pressure, and I could pass out. Eventually over the course of a year of trial and error, three medicines were found to help. Ten years later, a doctor in California weaned me off of these and changed me over to three different medicines that worked quite well.

During this most recent transaction, I was told to keep taking Aldactone (only repeat of the medicines tried in Mass General Hospital), which is a hormone diuretic, but only one a day instead of the three I had been taking. I asked him why I should take this one pill, and his comment was, "Most of the time a person is given medicines to lower their blood pressure and the pressure goes down. However, there is a gland on the kidney that controls certain aspects of blood pressure. After a time it recognizes that the blood pressure has changed since last it controlled it, so it takes an action to bring the blood pressure back to where the gland was controlling it before. The diuretic action of Aldactone is to keep the gland on the kidney busy so it won't push the blood pressure back up." Evidently he was right. The point is, the other two medicines he gave me had nothing to do with the kidney gland—one controlled my heart rate and the other was a beta-blocker.

However, now that the genome is "known," studies will lead to information about how the various genes work and which share duties with other genes. Having the genome on a computer allows one to agitate one gene and see if there is a response elsewhere in the system. The interplay will provide valuable information about how the body's immune system works. Since each person is different in some way, doctors will be able to compare the codes of a group of people that have a given disease against a group of people that do not have the disease. Then they will compare what is common to the diseased group and what isn't common on the disease-free group's code. This should lead them to a faster resolution of what it is that causes the disease. This would be fantastic information, since we know that the immune system works throughout the body. It reacts when you get a prick from a needle, and it works when a pathogen enters the body. It should be able to show us how the pathogen gets past the immune system and causes a disease that requires an antibiotic or some other response. Cause and effect is easier to study with a computer model containing the human genome. This is another wonder of life.

# HIV and AIDS—How They Relate to DNA and RNA

When reviewing earlier the various diseases and ailments that man has endured, I didn't include HIV (human immunodeficiency virus) and AIDS (acquired immunodeficiency syndrome) because of the nature of this disease. I felt that it was important for the reader to have a firm understanding of human DNA and RNA before reviewing the HIV virus and the related AIDS. These terrible diseases work almost like DNA and RNA, but in reverse. I talk about them separately, but they are both related.

A person acquires HIV before it turns into AIDS. In fact, the time from infection by HIV till a person is hit with AIDS is from two weeks to twenty years ... or forever. On average, a person has the HIV virus for ten years before it degenerates into full-blown AIDS. You will be able to realize why this takes so long as we describe the method by which one acquires HIV and it eventually becomes full-blown AIDS. It is important to realize I wrote this before methods in the past decade have been developed to keep some cases of HIV from degenerating into AIDS.

Realizing that AIDS may not show up for ten years gives you a feeling of why it was so hard to track down what was happening when AIDS first began its assault on mankind. In the early 1980s, people began to arrive at medical facilities around the world with symptoms that were like flu, or a bad cold, or pneumonia, and with sores and sicknesses that normally are more an irritant and not so persistent. Doctors found they could not relieve the symptoms with normal medications and treatments.

The fact that it appeared in various parts of the world at about the same time and with the same dire effects resulted in a great amount of research in looking for the cause of this pandemic. The first thing that made the sickness hard to isolate was that antibodies weren't found in the victims. Usually with the types of illness that were showing up, a medical exam would identify antibodies that the body generates to counteract the invader. The medical people and bio scientists test for antibodies; by identifying the antibody they can determine the antigen. After much time and research, the doctors that were in charge of this type of research in the United States and France began to believe that the illness was caused by a retrovirus. (58) A retrovirus can remain in the body in an inactive role for a long length of time before having an effect. There is another problem that prevailed at the time of this invasion, as I remember reading in the paper at the time.

A retrovirus possesses an RNA-type system as opposed to a human DNA genome. People can carry the HIV virus for days or weeks or years before showing any signs of antibodies in their system. A retrovirus is made up of RNA that enters the person's system. It then invades the DNA by passing its RNA through the protective shell surrounding the nucleus. Remember how I discussed, with regard to a human, the messenger RNA's transcription of the DNA inside the nucleus and then the mRNA passing out of the nucleus? This works just the opposite. The RNA of this retrovirus passes through the nucleus shell into the nucleus. Then a reverse transcription changes it from RNA to DNA, and that new DNA becomes a part of the person's DNA genome. This is a defective DNA genome. It replicates just like the original DNA, so it spreads into all the cells of the body.

At the time this was thought to be a retrovirus, the scientists of France and the United States worked long and hard to determine the culprit. Each found the result at about the same time through different techniques. It was difficult to pinpoint using normal medical techniques because in most cases the DNA of an infected individual was not reviewed.

Years before, there had been another outbreak of a sickness in San Francisco, in the late 1960s or early 1970s. The head doctor who was in charge of the identification program for our country, Dr. Robert Gallo, called to see if the doctors in San Francisco had any samples of blood from that earlier event. They did, and they forwarded them to Washington, DC. A review of the blood showed that indeed there was evidence of the same problem. However, in this case the antibodies were in the blood. Finally it was diagnosed by bio scientists in the United States and in France, and it was determined to be a retrovirus that invades the person's genetic material. Additional information at the time determined that this was a retrovirus that entered the system of a person through various rough sex acts; it was given various names, but finally the acronym AIDS—acquired immunodeficiency syndrome—stuck. (59) The individual who acquired this disease acquired it through some misdemeanor of their own. It wasn't just a random disease that hit based on statistics, but it hit specific people in the various countries due to stretching the sex act too far. It was later determined that HIV is transmitted by infected body fluids. This included using needles previously used by others with the infection. Dope addicts were transmitters of this disease by injecting dope into an HIV-infected body and then using the same needle to inject others. It was found that AIDS is transmitted by fluid transfer such as when a person is being operated on and a transfusion of blood is used. At the time blood banks were not screening the blood for this retrovirus. The original source of AIDS appeared to be through male homosexual sex acts. This, initially, was identified as the main cause of the disease, because the sex acts between two males were quite violent in nature. Anal sex acts could result in the tearing of the tissues and bleeding. For this reason the gay community in the United States showed the effects of this problem early. Recent information indicates that the first carrier of this disease came from Haiti in 1969. So this probably started the sickness that sometimes takes ten years to show up. As time passed, the HIV disease in the United States and other developed countries became prevalent in females also and eventually in newborn children who were infected by the disease.

As indicated, the HIV virus enters the person's system. He may not even show symptoms. In many cases infected persons don't realize they are infected and continue having sex. A person can carry HIV without any signs of infection for as long as ten to twenty years. Some people are actually immune to this disease due to some characteristic of their genome and other body functions. However, eventually, in most cases the HIV and the subsequent AIDS hits the person and hits them hard.

One of the other major factors relates to people using drugs that they inject using other people's needles. If the other person has HIV, it can be transferred via the needle into the person's blood. Since this mode of infection was brought to the world's attention, some locations in the United States and other countries have programs where they supply needles to drug users, so that they will not continue the practice of using infected needles. This program has helped. Another major cause was due to transfusions. Since this retrovirus was unknown and wasn't easy to find, blood donated by people with HIV would be used in operations on people who had no risk factors for this disease, and they would end up suffering through no fault of their own. An African American tennis star, Arthur Ashe of the United States, was operated on for some minor problem and acquired the disease from tainted blood and eventually died of AIDS. This brought the problem to a high visibility because of Arthur Ashe's popularity.

The main issue at the time was learning how to screen for the problem, especially finding a way of reviewing blood in the blood banks to determine the purity of the blood. The doctors had to find the virus so they could take samples and try various techniques for finding and eliminating the sources of it. The problem was that there were no good ways to obtain enough of the virus to work with. I remember reading twenty-five years ago about how they solved a part of this problem. The doctor in charge of the US program, Robert Gallo, was trying to determine the nature of the disease and a possible cure, but he couldn't find how to get enough samples to work with. He and his assistants were not successful in finding a way to generate a significant number of the pathogens. Gallo had to leave to attend a conference in France concerning the subject matter. The French had done considerable work on this issue, and it was hoped that the combined inputs from each would result in a plan of attack. Gallo left instructions with his lab assistants to try to find ways to generate enough of the virus so they could do battle with it. After Gallo left and they began to work on a method for generating large numbers of the HIV virus, the male technician remembered some effects he had seen on people with leukemia. He decided to try an experiment where he used this leukemia blood as the soup for the small sample he had of the HIV virus. The two prepared a broth of the leukemia blood and the HIV virus and placed it in an incubator to keep the temperature constant. By the time they came back the next day and reviewed the results, they were shocked to see an enormous amount of the live virus on the microscope slide. They were excited by the results, but they didn't want to contact Dr. Gallo in France and excite him over something that may have just been a bit of good fortune. Gallo was a stickler on details and exact results, and they didn't want to disturb him while he was in conference.

So they decided to try again. They set up the culture and had another go at it, and the next day they had the same results. They then decided to contact Gallo. They sent him a telegram, and he got word in France that they had had some success. He finished some immediate things he had to do and then flew back to Washington, DC. He went directly to the lab where his technicians had set things up again, because they knew he was so thorough that he would have to see for himself. They discussed their method and what the results were, and, sure enough, he wanted to see for himself. The next day the look through the microscope showed they had found the right recipe. Gallo was surprised by this rapid result from his two assistants. This now provided a method for producing enough of the virus to work on. It was under this framework that more was learned about the virus and how to screen for it in the blood held in the blood banks. Ever since that time, advances by bio scientists have provided methods for screening of blood. Problems with the blood bank supplies have been very rare in developed societies over the last twenty years. During the 1980s and 1990s, many people would have a pint of their own blood set aside every six months and stored for any future problems that might occur … such as the need for an operation where they might need blood transfusions. Although this was a good idea for those wealthy enough to afford it, it was no longer needed as the blood banks became reliable.

When a retrovirus becomes part of a person's genome and is stored in the DNA of his or her chromosomes, it can be passed on to the next generation. The pregnancy of a woman results, as we have discussed, in a chromosome that is some mixture of the chromosomes of the two individuals involved. This means the DNA of the child may be infected. These are called endogenous retroviruses. Of an estimated 2.8 million lives lost to AIDS in 2005, 570,000 were children as a result of this scenario.

Sub-Saharan Africa remains by far the worst affected region, with an estimated 21.6 to 27.4 million people currently living with HIV. (61) Approximately two million of them are children under fifteen years of age. More than 64 percent of all people living with HIV are in sub-Saharan Africa, as are more than three-quarters of all women living with HIV. In 2005, there were between 10.6 and 13.6 million AIDS orphans living in sub-Saharan Africa.

South and Southeast Asia are the second-worst affected regions, with 15 percent of the total. AIDS accounts for the deaths of 500,000 children in this region annually. Two-thirds of HIV and AIDS infections in Asia occur in India, with 9.4 million (0.9 percent of population), surpassing South Africa's estimated 4.9 to 6.1 million (11.9 percent of population) infections, making India the country with the highest number of HIV infections in the world. (34) In the thirty-five African nations with the highest prevalence, average life expectancy is 48.3 years—6.5 years less than it would be without the disease. [61]

There is no cure for HIV. There has been tremendous progress made in relieving the distress from this disease, especially in developed countries, where certain high-priced drugs are available. Because reverse transcription lacks the usual proofreading of DNA replication, this kind of virus mutates very often. This enables the virus to quickly grow resistant to antiviral pharmaceuticals and impedes the development of an effective vaccine against the retrovirus HIV. Two of the places in the body that become major targets for this disease are the tonsils and adenoids. I personally would recommend that, where medical treatment is available, young people have these removed. Perhaps the people affected with HIV should also have their tonsils and adenoids removed to at least eliminate this target area and reduce any discomfort in these areas.

There are other diseases that the HIV+ person can pass on other than HIV. People suffering from AIDS contract many other diseases due to their immune system's lack of response. Because of this, the victims may contract such diseases as tuberculosis, which could be passed on to a partner. Tuberculosis can be treated and cured, but it's not an easy battle. Acquired immunodeficiency syndrome results in damage to the immune system that cannot be reversed. As the virus works its bad medicine on the immune system, the victims are hit with infections of all sorts. There are terrible flu-like symptoms, pneumonia or pneumonia-like symptoms, tumors, rashes, sores, breathing problems, eyesight problems—and the list goes on.

The only good thing about AIDS is that people without AIDS are now aware of how powerful their immune system must be to be able to counter and to keep all these illnesses at bay. The natural immunity that a body builds up is tremendous. People think they can't get rid of a cold, but they do. Once a cold has hit and the body builds up its immunity and the cold is conquered, the virus that caused that cold will not cause one any longer in the future. However, there are many viruses that cause colds, so they keep coming, especially in the winter each year. (People don't suffer from many of these illnesses in the Southern Hemisphere where it is warm. There are much fewer illnesses like colds and flu. In fact, the word *flu* comes from the word *influenza,* which means "during cold weather.") Time after time, a person gets colds as he grows older. Many people at ages above fifty-five find themselves free of the colds they used to get. It's because they are immune to many strains, and they no longer have children bringing the new strains home from school. So that is probably one advantage of old age.

Treatments for AIDS and HIV exist to decelerate the virus's progression in its victim, but with no known cure. Recent work has shown an approach to prevent HIV and even solve it. The word is out as to how to prevent AIDS. The HIV virus is transmitted through bodily fluids, such as through anal, vaginal, or oral sex; blood contact to exposed wounds to the body; blood transfusions; contaminated hypodermic needles; and these types of blood exposures. The best method to avoid the problem is not to have sex with anyone that is known to have the problem. The next best thing is not to have sex with someone you don't know or haven't known long enough to know his or her sex habits. There are steps to be taken to prevent exposure even if the sex partner is not known well enough, such as the use of condoms by men and condoms made for women. Although not perfect, barrier methods are estimated to be 90+ percent perfect. In cases where consistent and correct use of condoms is maintained, couples where one partner is infected show that the HIV infection rate for the uninfected partner is less than 1 percent. Women are taught to carry condoms in case the opportunity arises and the male doesn't carry condoms. Women that happen to be promiscuous wear a rubber diaphragm inside their vagina and dispose or clean it after any intercourse. Being faithful is a strong course of action. This mostly applies to the male member of the marriage or partnership, who is normally the one that feels the urge and doesn't want to take the time to put on a condom.

The use of clean needles and methods to ensure zero risk has changed in hospitals as well as by drug addicts. Different methods for extracting the needles to be used for a blood sample are not as casual as they once were. Needles are discarded religiously in the medical areas. Rubber gloves are worn in more places. A scratch occurring on a nurse is treated immediately. In basketball games if a player is injured and bleeds, he is removed from the game until the problem is corrected. I find that this scourge that has come in the form of HIV has resulted in techniques to prevent the spread of the disease and, probably more importantly, provided a higher level of hygiene throughout the medical and nonmedical communities that did not prevail before this problem. This is probably the most encouraging progress, since it helps for all diseases, not just for HIV. There are additional steps taken, such as mothers who have HIV are told not to breast-feed their child so as not to pass on this problem via this fluid.

UNAIDS and the World Health Organization estimate that AIDS has killed more than twenty-five million people since it was first recognized in 1981, making it one of the most destructive epidemics in recorded history. Despite recent improved access to antiretroviral treatment and care in many regions of the world, the AIDS epidemic claimed an estimated 2.8 million lives in 2005. Globally, between 33.4 and 46 million people in 2015 live with HIV. In 2005, between 3.4 and 6.2 million people were newly infected, and between 2.4 and 3.3 million people with AIDS died, an increase from 2003 and the highest number since 1981. (59)

The development of highly active antiretroviral therapy (HAART) as effective therapy for HIV infection and AIDS has substantially reduced the death rate from this disease in those areas where these drugs are widely available. This has created the misperception that the disease has vanished. In fact, as the life expectancy of persons with AIDS has increased in countries where HAART is widely used, the number of persons living with AIDS has increased substantially. In the United States, the number of persons with AIDS increased from about 35,000 in 1988 to 220,000 in 1996. The life expectancy of those that are treated has increased to 32.2 years. In the absence of antiretroviral therapy, the median time of progression from HIV infection to AIDS is nine to ten years, and the median survival time after one develops AIDS is only nine months. (59)

There was a recent short article in the New Yorker section of the *Wall Street Journal* by Michael Specter entitled, "A Look Back May Push AIDS Fight Ahead," which I thought was applicable to the subject I am covering here.

"The body's past battles against retroviruses such as HIV having been a major engine of evolution and perhaps lies behind some of the most important steps in human development," writes Michael Specter.

Scientists are gaining these insights by reconstructing extinct forms of retroviruses. Retroviruses reproduce by imprinting parts of themselves onto a cell's DNA. In some cases, this means they become a part of a species' DNA. The damaged remnants of retroviruses make up about 8 percent of the human genome. Many of those viral fragments are shared with chimpanzees and monkeys.

Scientists around the world have recently been reconstructing the original viruses from these fragments, careful to ensure the reborn diseases are able to reproduce themselves only once.

This has been sufficient to show the role retroviruses have played in human development. For instance, they seem to have led mammals to form a placenta, which makes it possible to produce offspring with larger brains than egg-laying animals.

Another reconstructed virus might provide a clue as to why HIV, which infects chimpanzees as easily as it does humans, doesn't harm these animals.

A recent experiment showed that humans have developed an effective defense against an extinct retrovirus, called PtERV (pronounced "pea-terv"). Chimpanzees haven't. The experiment suggested that this lack of a defense against one retrovirus actually makes chimpanzees immune to the effects of another, HIV.

This approach is still decades away from creating a cure for AIDS, Mr. Specter says, but already has suggested new lines of attack.

These types of experiments going on all over the world are bringing a learning curve to the scientists trying to find a cure for AIDS or a means of preventing the virus.

The impact of AIDS on the world is evident when one looks at the median ages of the various countries of the world. The median age in Africa is nineteen years, which is the youngest of any continent. The country with the lowest median age in the world is also found on the African continent: Uganda. The landlocked east African nation of Uganda has a median age of fifteen years, meaning that half the country's population is younger than fifteen years old and half is older. In contrast, Mauritius, an island off east Africa, with a median age of thirty-one years, has the highest average in Africa. (59)

The median age in India, the world's second most populous country, is twenty-four. In comparison, the median age in China is much higher, at thirty-four years.

## HIV and AIDS Are Hard to Get!

It's important that the reader understands that HIV and AIDS are impossible to contract. What do I mean by that? I mean just as I say. Humans have to go out of their way to get AIDS. With proper attention, HIV and the resultant AIDS is very hard to acquire. You can't get it from kissing, even though there's an exchange of fluids in this act. You can't get it from tears in the eyes from one to another. You can't get it from the doorknobs of men's or women's bathroom facilities. If people with these two diseases leave a bathroom facility after relieving themselves or having masturbated and put their hands on the doorknob, you won't get HIV or AIDS if you place your hand on that doorknob. You won't get it from the commode seat in the bathroom. You won't contract HIV from urine. The HIV virus is very weak under normal conditions. The HIV virus cannot retain its potential under normal living conditions, such as being exposed to everyday air. It doesn't lie around waiting to infect a person like some bacteria do. Chances are you won't even get it from semen from a person unless it involves sexual intercourse that is rough in nature. The biggest risks come from blood transfusions in those countries or areas where blood is not screened or there is a transfusion directly from a person who has the disease. From direct transfusion from a person with the disease, the estimated risk is 90 percent. Childbirth by an infected mother has a 25 percent risk. From here, the risk factor drops to less than 1 percent for the widely distributed list of potential sources, such as oral sex and anal sex—less than 1 percent out of ten thousand incidents.

So what does this mean? It means that after study of this disease for about twenty-five years, the data show it is hard to acquire HIV and the related AIDS. It is not contagious. It is not like any other disease that you might think about and worry about contracting, diseases like cancer, tuberculosis, influenza, infection, *Staphylococcus*, pneumonia, *Streptococcus*, malaria, and many other diseases that may come your way no matter how well you live. It's not like other illnesses that are a function of your age and cause heart failure, or hardening of the arteries, or liver failure and those things that eventually will happen to each of us if we live long enough. Having any of these normal illnesses when and if they come your way is a matter of statistics, your basic health, where you live, surgery, heredity, accidents that lead to other complications, your environment, and so on. You will die from something.

However, you will not get HIV and the eventual AIDS no matter what, as long as you live a natural, healthy life away from unprotected sex—at least in this country. You can't get it from breathing right next to a person with AIDS. If you could, there would be many doctors and nurses in this world with the infection. It's almost impossible to acquire HIV if you live a normal life. AIDS is what it says it is—acquired immunodeficiency. You have to go out of your way to acquire HIV and the resultant AIDS.

### Recent Advances on HIV and AIDS

There have been some dramatic recent advances on preventing HIV from becoming AIDS. There have also been advances on increasing the time between HIV and AIDS. There are very detailed reports concerning these advances, and one should go to Google or Firefox on one's computer to read the details. This would take another book beyond this one, so I will leave that research up to the reader. I can say that they have found combinations of drugs that enable two major advances: one, a combination that takes the HIV and prevents the development of the AIDS virus for many years and perhaps forever in some people; and two, a combination that allows people with AIDS to suffer much less and live an almost normal life.

# Ebola –
# Another Contagious Disease

Ebola has been around for centuries, and every so often there is a small outbreak of this disease.

In 2014 there was a major outbreak in northwestern Africa. Three countries have been affected dramatically—Liberia, Ghana, and Sierra Leone—with high infection levels of people and about a 50 percent death rate of those affected. Several countries, including the United States, have been hurriedly working on a vaccine to transfer to these countries. A vaccine was developed in mid-January 2015 that worked on mice and was shipped to Liberia by the end of January 2015. Recent results indicate this vaccine is effective in most cases.

The key element to date on this outbreak is to isolate these countries' travel outside their country. They are essentially under quarantine isolation. People flying from one of these countries must pass a medical check to ensure they don't have the symptoms of this disease. This disease is like HIV virus in that one must make physical contact with the person carrying the disease in a direct manner. It is hard to pass on. Even so, American doctors working on patients—even though they were properly clothed to prevent their bodies from making contact and wore special breathing equipment to prevent taking in the fumes from the area or patients—have returned to this country and had the early symptoms of the disease. They were quarantined and handled with special practices for a month before they were pronounced free of the disease. To date no American has been shown to have the full Ebola disease.

# Status of Actions Taken to Prevent Reoccurrence of the Five Major Elements of Death

I previously described the five major causes of death that occurred in the fourteenth and nineteenth centuries. Here we are in the twenty-first century, and we can review what actions have been taken to prevent reoccurrences of these dramatic elements.

### The Great Famine—Status as of January 2015

There have been two major factors to prevent a reoccurrence of the Great Famine:

Industrial Revolution—The Industrial Revolution began around 1850. This was a revolution of the way things were performed prior to 1850 and what occurred after that date. Several pieces of major equipment for the production of food were established. First came electricity, and this was the prime mover of the development of motors. Oil wells were installed in Pennsylvania, which provided the power for running motors and generators. Within a short time equipment like motor-driven plows was introduced along with automatic feeders of fields of food plants like corn and wheat. The reaping of huge fields of things such as corn or wheat was done by power-driven machines rather than by hand. With electricity came electric lights that allowed for work around the clock; previously much farmwork was done from early in the morning till it got dark. This made available a greater production capability of all foods. Invention after invention occurred to provide the greater production of food all over the world. Along with the ability to provide much more food, there were the means of transporting those foods, such as the oil-driven train, the car, the airplane, and huge transport ships; as time progressed, these means of transportation were improved to make things happen more rapidly. Refrigeration allowed for longer storage times between the times crops or animal food was made available till it was transported; an increase in storage also took place. World trade began with the help of these pieces of equipment. Crops of certain foods that were not grown in parts of the world received them from other countries with the increase in transportation. The world became alive with production from many means that were developed. Better methods of selection of the seeds and other means of improving the initial elements used to plant crops of all types were developed. Productivity became better year after year as long as the weather remained satisfactory. Poor weather in some areas limited that area's production for a year, but other areas of the world produced more to keep things positive.

North and South America—Keep in mind that the Great Famine occurred in the fourteenth century and the world didn't know about the existence of "the New World"—North and South America—at that time. They didn't come along until the seventeenth century. From the countries such as the United States came new crops never heard of in Europe and the rest of the world. There was corn being grown by the Indians of America, and this eventually provided the whole world with a source of a new food—a food that could be grown in many countries later in the following centuries. Turkeys were found in America and eventually became one of the major food sources of the meat eaters of the world. The weather in these two continents saw areas that were ideal for growing fruits and vegetables and large herds of cattle unlike any other country of the world. There were ample water supplies for most of these areas for providing large crops. Countries like the United States and Brazil had huge areas of undeveloped land that could be used for such things as grazing of huge herds of cattle. Not only were there new food types for the world to consume, but probably more important, the United States produced crops and meat foods that could supply the world, since the production was greater than what could be consumed by the US population. Along with the new foods and greater productivity, the advancement of bigger and faster airplanes allowed for the transportation of these resources all over the world. The advancement of bigger and faster oceangoing ships allowed for large shipments around the world from North and South America.

These two sources of food made worldwide famine disappear. There are times when production is down for certain foods due to weather or other means, but it usually only causes a rise in the cost of production followed by increases of the price until production is back to normal.

As the population of the world grows from seven billion people in 2015 to ten billion in the future, there may be a problem due to this large increase in population and demand for more food. However, I believe as the world grows older and the population bigger, there will be breakthroughs in several things, such as new sources of energy. There also will be improved diets developed that the world's population will thrive on. Change will cause change, but man has always found a way to persist.

### The Black Death—Status as of 2015

It took several hundred years for us to understand what caused the Black Death, which is caused by the bites of fleas from a certain type of rat. Back in the fourteenth century there was very limited communication around the world to spread the word to eliminate this rat and isolate people that have this disease. As I previously mentioned, in the fourteenth century there were no printers or other means of rapid communication. Now let's look at what the world is like in 2015.

Mass communication—today finds communication that is unbelievable compared to just a few decades ago. We have computers, the Internet, iPhones (and other phones), iPads (and other forms of this means of communication) that can spread the word around the world in seconds. If two people die from a disease, this news is spread around the world, as well as the possible cause. The world is sensitized to begin isolation as rapidly as possible of the people showing up with the disease, and a minute-by-minute reports are seen concerning that given disease. Examples of this relate recently to a flu that is different than the virus the flu shots have prepared the world's population to deal with. The word got out to place people with this flu in isolation from others. The flu is spread through the air by people with the flu breathing and spitting and coughing. Since a person is the spreader, the odds go up for people to catch the flu if they are in crowds of people; so the word goes out to stay away from crowded places. People with this flu are even kept from some hospitals so the hospitals don't become a big source of the problem. In hospitals that regularly handle flu, they keep the patients only a short time and send them home and tell them not to go to school for a week or so. The point is, we try to isolate the sick from the healthy and take these actions as soon as is practical.

For another good example of why the Black Death, or a medical problem like this, should not reach the levels it did in the fourteenth century, one only has to look at how the Ebola disease in northwest Africa is presently being handled. People in the three main countries where this is prevalent are restricted in moving from one country to another. People that are there visiting relatives are not allowed to board airplanes to return or go to other parts of the world without passing certain medical tests. In other words, people and countries are being quarantined. The medical teams from the United States are provided with special clothing to prevent direct contact with patients as well as special breathing apparatus to prevent their breathing in the air while attending patients. Doctors returning to the United States must past certain medical tests and in some cases are put into isolation or quarantined. In essence we are trying to restrict those countries from spreading the Ebola virus. There are checks on people traveling to and from those countries not only when they are boarding planes but also when they eventually are disembarking from those planes.

While all of this is proceeding, there are doctors in various countries in the world working on potential vaccines against the Ebola virus. A recent article in the paper described how a potential vaccine that has been generated in the United States is proceeding to Liberia to try on control groups. As I previously mentioned results indicate the vaccine works. Wouldn't this be a miracle if this worked after having had this problem exist in Europe and other parts of the world six hundred years ago? This would answer the question about what the world would do if the Black Death appeared again. We would put our latest technologies to work as we did on Ebola and overcome the issue rapidly. It seems we need catastrophes to bring out the best in us.

It is important that there has been much progress from the last few months of 2014 through the first two months of 2015, and the Ebola disease in the three countries of Africa has dropped considerably. This progress was mainly achieved through restricted travel, better knowledge, and the communication of events in the countries involved, and mainly through isolation of those with the disease from those that have proved to be strong enough to avoid it. Restrictions are involved as a medical approach is awaited. Perhaps the main good thing about this recent Ebola bout has been the procedures that worked and perhaps the ability to try out new vaccines that work against the disease. If a vaccine is found, we can begin to treat this disease as we have other diseases in the past—and win (looks like 2015 will be the year).

Keep in mind that many of the people that died during the Black Death and Great Famine died from pneumonia that developed as a result of those factors. Today, people get pneumonia shots to prevent or alleviate any pneumonia-type problems. The shots are especially given to young people and older people who are more susceptible to pneumonia.

Medicine in general has improved, as indicated in my discussions. There were little or no medical factors to help people during those two bad periods. Thanks to better living conditions, antibiotics, better sanitation, and better habits, there were approximately two thousand cases in 2003 worldwide

Approximately ten to twenty people in the United States develop the plague each year, primarily from prairie dogs in rural areas of the Southwest, with approximately a 15 percent dying. There has not been a person-to-person infection in the United States since 1924.

## *The Flu Pandemic—Status as of 2015*

While there were some methods to handle flu in 1918, they were only able to handle it superficially. The flu first hit in the first few months of 1918 and caused a normal three to five days of flu fever, and rest and drinking fluids were all that was required. This affected the normal sector of the population—young children and older adults. The flu that hit late in 1918 and caused the major death problems was a flu that was not understood at the time. It was years before it was realized that the deaths from the flu in the later part of 1918 were caused by the strong immune systems of the normally healthy individuals who were consumed by this problem within days. Essentially, the early flu of 1918 allowed the normally strong individuals that were between twenty and forty-five years old to establish a level of immunity that kept them from getting flu. The flu bug that came back in late 1918 was met by this increased immunity by this older and stronger group of people. Their immune systems had already built up an immunity level from the early 1918 flu. These normally healthy and strong individuals with their, at this time, abnormally strong immune systems were so strong they literally ate up the flu and ravished the body cells of these groups of people, and they died within days. This had never been seen before and to my knowledge was never seen again.

One must keep in mind that this flu hit as World War I was ending. It is believed that many of the deaths due to flu were due to the weakened systems of those who had spent a great deal of time in trenches during the war. They were weak, and some had relatively low cases of other diseases such as pneumonia or heavy cold symptoms when the flu hit. It is noted that most of the flu's victims were in the battle zones of Europe in World War I. The death rate was much higher in Europe than in the United States, Canada, or South America. In addition, living conditions at the end of the war were not conducive to good health or good health practices. I don't expect these conditions to prevail at this time.

Today we know of various types of flu strains and methods that were developed to prevent flu in general. There is one important thing to remember: if people get flu from one strain of the flu, they are essentially immune from that strain. This proved to be the means of overcoming flu in general. The body's immune system is a wondrous thing; once it builds up antibodies for a given strain of the flu, it is buried in its immune system forever and it will be immune to this strain. This turns out to be true for many bacterial and viral infections such as measles and polio.

There are basically three strains of the flu bug that are common around the world to people. As people get older and have had flu several times in their life, they are in pretty good shape to not get flu again, or if they do it is less severe. They build up some resistance to the three basic types:

H1N1—prevalent in California and the states close by; called influenza A or just A.

H3N2—prevalent in Texas and areas around Texas; called influenza A also.

Type B—found more in the Northeast states; called influenza B. There are at least two types of flu B.

Vaccines for the flu are determined each year based on selected data on the ones that are circulating and how they compare to past strains. If they are similar, how well did the vaccine work?

There are about 150 influenza centers around the world, and they are continually reviewed by the world's countries. In addition, they send the viruses to the five WHO organizations that are located in Australia, Japan, England, and China. This information is the prime information for determining what viruses will be selected for immunization shots. Although WHO sends the information around the world to all countries with their recommended strains for the flu shots, different countries determine what they will use. In many cases certain countries will not use the recommendations, since they have information that they believe is more pertinent for their location.

The flu vaccine is grown from the clinical recommended strains and the country's prior experience. Timing is quite important, since it takes approximately six months for the vaccine to be generated with the selected virus information. The virus is grown in healthy selected chicken species in January of the year, since it takes six months to generate the virus and the vaccine in time for the flu season, which arrives in the United States in October/November. Of course it arrives at different times in other countries of the world. Vaccines help people develop immunity by imitation an infection. Once the imitation of the flu has been in the body for approximately ten days, the body has developed antibodies and its immune system is left with these forever.

And then comes the flu season, and each country begins to analyze the species and how effective the vaccine will be against what they find. This past year there was an additional strain found that was not included with the vaccine—only later data will tell how well the vaccine worked without this strain being included. Medical people say that what is in the vaccine and what the immune system has had in its history will determine the success of the vaccine. It is believed that even if people don't possess the vaccine against one of the strains in this year's flu, they will probably not have a significant illness due to the body being somewhat protected due to similarity.

If the vaccine contains flu species that are common to the flu that is going around in a flu season, it is said there is a "good match"; if it is like this season, it is called a "mismatch." We will have to see how well the body responds to this mismatched vaccine. We will know as the months move on from the beginning of this year's season through to May of 2015. Most of the vaccines provided in the past have proved to be at least effective against a "mismatch" in that victims didn't suffer as much as would be expected. As mentioned, it is important that the people who are infected have had one kind of flu or more during their lifetime and have had flu shots for the last seventy years, and one of them may have proved to help at this time.

Some strains of the flu virus do not grow well in eggs. This is true of the H3N2 virus strain, and medical firms are working to find ways to improve this vaccine. Some firms are working on other ways to provide the proper vaccine.

Although a great amount of time and energy are supplied around the world, the fact that it takes six months to generate a vaccine means there is six months when a new species pops up; that's life.

It is strongly recommended that people wash their hands and face often during the flu season. This is especially true when people have been around a crowd of people and return home. Still, the best way to prevent the flu is to get a flu shot and wash yourself after being around a crowd of people. There is no doubt that the flu has been greatly reduced since the advent of the flu shot.

### World Wars I and II—Status as of 2015

Why should we expect that there won't be a World War III? Keep in mind that World War I and World War II were caused by two countries—Germany and Japan—with Germany causing both wars in Europe while Japan started the war in Asia and the United States. These two countries were greatly industrialized—better than any other two countries. The Germans wanted all the land of Europe and were the most powerful country in Europe. It didn't help that Hitler came along, and much of the war was caused by his ambitions. In Japan the Second World War was started in China because Japan was running out of land for producing rice and other foods. So their initial move was to invade Southeast Asia in the hope of gaining large pieces of land for growing rice. Their initial success and their large, powerful navy made them feel more powerful, and they believed that there was no country or no reason for not entering into a war. At the same time, with Germany's success in Europe, they felt the United States would be in no position to handle both the European war and war with them. They felt if they could destroy the US Pacific fleet that they would be free to invade and conquer any of the island nations in the Pacific.

With these situations being a fact and the loss of the wars by Germany (twice) in Europe and Japan in the Pacific the first level of control to prevent World War III was to control these countries. This level of control by the United States, the United Kingdom, France, and Russia is meant to provide early indications of any possible repeat events.

In Europe after World War II, the Allies had commanding positions and governments in both East and West Germany. Germany was to demilitarize, and they were limited in their production of fighter airplanes and other military-type weapons. Half of Berlin was controlled by Russia (called East Berlin) and the other half by England and the United States (the Western Allies) and called West Berlin. These were effective for many years ... but what about the rest of the world?

Why not any other countries? Keep in mind that the United States had dropped two atomic bombs to end the war in the Pacific with Japan. Keep in mind that no other country had this major capability for several years. It was obvious that this type of weapon allowed the United States to command respect around the world and this prevented the next big war, but what about other countries developing this capability?

Sure enough, by 1949 Russia had developed an atomic bomb. In 1952 the United Kingdom had the capability. In 1960 France had the capability and China in 1964. Later India and Pakistan had nuclear reactor power. By 1953 a hydrogen bomb was in Russia's weapons list. Why worry about Russia, since it had been one of our allies during the past war? Well, it so happens when a country like Russia gets something that puts them "on top of the world," so to speak, they begin to feel their oats and start making loud noises like they want to do something; so a "Cold War" began between Russia and the United States. It was called this since no bombing-type war was started—just a war of words and trying to outdo each other. Still, there were no major threats of an atomic war between the two countries.

## *Then Came the Intercontinental Missiles*

Russia (USSR) worked and progressed on developing missiles that could carry an atomic bomb. Their first successful one was in May of 1957 and could hit targets about 250 miles away. No worry by the United States, since they had a great fleet of ships and eventually submarines that could launch missiles almost anywhere in the world. The first successful atomic missile by the United States was in November of 1958. The United States was behind the Soviets until President John F. Kennedy made it a priority item with a program called "the Apollo Program," which used the Saturn rocket technology funded by President Eisenhower. This proved to be successful and was used for space systems. Since they proved their ability to fly into outer space, it became obvious that they could be programmed to hit any country in the world. Russia and the United States had this capability of hitting anyplace in the world. These systems being used as intercontinental missile systems were outlawed by a 1971 ABM treaty.

By the 1960s it was assumed there would be as many as thirty to thirty-five countries with nuclear weapons. It turns out that most of the countries looked at the five countries that had huge capabilities, knowing they would not be able to catch up. They deemed it necessary to take steps so the ones that did possess this awful capability would come to some form of agreement that would satisfy those countries— that the five countries that did have large nuclear capabilities would find a way to agree among themselves to a worldwide control. This started the various countries working toward a safe world.

In 1972 the SALT treaty froze the number of ICBM launchers that the Soviets and the United States possessed and allowed new submarines with SLM launchers only if an equal number of land-based ICBM launchers were dismantled.

In 1991 the United States and the Soviet Union agreed with the START I treaty to reduce their deployable ICBMs and their related warheads. This was the beginning of the end of the Cold War.

By the year 2009 the five nations that have ICBM capability were on the United Nations Security Council. This gave great strength toward the future peace of the world.

It is of note that all the ICBM capabilities of the five countries that have ICBMs improved them with multiple independently deployable warheads, allowing each of the warheads to hit different targets. All systems are much smaller but better controlled through things such as integrated circuits. (I am proud to say I personally made, during my lunch hours, the first silicon integrated circuit in the world on a single chip in 1959.)

In 1980 the International Atomic Energy Agency (IAEA) was established with the purpose of providing a safeguard system under the Nuclear Non-Proliferation Treaty (NPT), which has been successful to date in curbing the diversion of uranium by countries into military uses. Even though there are countries such as India that have nuclear reactor capability, they use it to construct nuclear reactors for the purpose of generating electricity. Nuclear reactors process uranium to a 20 percent purity, which is not capable of making an explosive device. To make an explosive device, the uranium must be processed to 80 percent purity. Under the various treaties it is legal to transport uranium from one country to the next with the stipulation that it cannot be purified to the 80 percent purity level; and this has been respected by the various countries. There are several concerns that Iran, for one, is trying to purify uranium they possess to the 80 percent level. Iran is suspected of this but denies it; however, they will not allow any other country representatives into their facilities to witness their levels of processing. As this is written the United States has been negotiating with Iran to allow inspections of their processing. This negotiation has been recently extended for another six months. If nothing is resolved in this time frame, it is expected that several countries will take more forceful actions to preserve world safety.

In general, there is no major world war seen in the near future. The precautions taken with the various NPT and IAEA treaties have stabilized the nuclear situation with the countries of the world.

In summary, there is almost zero chance of the world having any of the five killers of life I listed, as a result of the actions that have occurred to prevent repeating these death threats. However, as we learn more about life as we know it, we can see the possibilities of other threats. The world gets older, related to the ages of those living. The life span is now over seventy-six in the United States, and there are other countries that have higher average life spans. Scientists and doctors the world over continue to investigate life's threats as we get older. Some people are born with insufficient insulin and suffer from sugar diabetes. This has been termed "type 1 diabetes." This has been overcome by their taking insulin on a daily basis, which they have to do for a lifetime. However, it has been noted that there are now many people that didn't have this problem, but due to foods or age or both now have what is termed type 2 diabetes. Type 2 diabetes is when the insulin the person has is not high enough to convert the higher level of sugar in their blood, and this is termed "high blood sugar." Today's people eat more foods that are high in sugar. The number of people that have this condition is rising rapidly. It is believed to be related to the fortunate living levels many of the world's people are presently living. Their more fortunate living level allows them to eat more of the foods they previously were denied for one reason or another; as they take in higher levels of processed foods, or even natural foods that have a high sugar content, they begin to show signs of a rise in their blood sugar. The actions taken are to reduce their weight by eating less food and specifically certain foods. They are directed to take in less processed foods that contain high levels of sugar and other chemicals that can contribute to this problem. They are directed to eat less red meat and especially those that have a high fat content. They are directed to eat more produce and eat somewhat like a vegetarian. They are directed to exercise to help burn off calories. By eating healthy, exercising, and losing body weight, they can reduce their blood sugar levels to a point where the insulin their body produces is satisfactory to provide a healthy body.

Why do I bring up the issue of type 2 diabetes? It's because the number of people diagnosed with this type of problem has increased dramatically and this is one of the signs that living to an older age and being able to afford richer foods can cause new problems. This is only one of the problems that the world's older population and better living conditions can cause. As the average life span increases, we will probably find other new problems that can be immense and relate to possible higher death rates. So we may avoid the five problems that have been discussed but come up with new issues that would cause a high level of deaths. The medical community knows this and continues to learn more about the human body and any new possible weaknesses that begin to show as we reach higher average life spans.

# Life and Life Span

The world population has experienced continuous growth since the end of the Great Famine and the Black Death in 1350, when it was near 370 million. The highest growth rates—global population increases above 1.8 percent per year—occurred briefly during the 1950s, and for longer periods during the 1960s and 1970s. The global growth rate peaked at 2.2 percent in 1963 and has declined to below 1.1 percent as of 2012. Total annual births were highest in the late 1980s at about 138 million, and are now expected to remain essentially constant at their 2011 level of 134 million, mainly due to controlled birth rates in several of the large countries of the world. Deaths presently number 56 million per year and are expected to increase to 80 million per year by 2040, mainly due to significant population growth while the death rate percentage is maintained. (5)

This improvement in the life span of people is taking place in the undeveloped countries (1). One of the biggest problems relates to countries, including the United States, that have control of diseases using the various vaccines installed to prevent bacterial and viral diseases, but stop using them properly. A measles epidemic of sorts is now proceeding in the United States, mainly due to the lack of everyone getting measles vaccine. What was once about 90 percent of children over six months of age, and young adults, getting measles vaccines have dropped in many states to 70 percent. Parents and young adults are deciding not to get vaccines. They had heard that youngsters get autism from these vaccines. This has been proved to be incorrect, but the parents still avoid getting their children vaccinated. This is unfair, since those not getting the vaccines are putting other people in danger. Measles is a virus and only requires a person with the virus in his or her system to be breathing out the virus. This is more likely to be spread if the person with the disease is in a crowd. The present outbreak is related to large crowds going to Disneyland recently, and some had the measles virus in their system.

## Viral Diseases—Controlled though Vaccines

The other viral diseases that are infectious but in some cases can be controlled are:

Hepatitis A, oral

Hepatitis B, saliva, mother's milk

Hepatitis C, blood, sexual contact

Herpes, saliva and lesions

HIV, sexual contact, blood, mother's milk

Influenza virus, droplets, breathing in a crowd where flu is prevalent

Mumps, droplets, contact

Polio, oral, crowd in a swimming pool

Rabies, animal bite, droplet contact

Rubella (German measles), droplet contact

## Bacterial Diseases—Controlled or Cured through Antibiotics

Anthrax, skin penetration, inhalation, through skin abrasions of spore-contaminated dust

Chlamydial pneumonia, respiratory droplets from a community

*Legionella*, called Legionnaires' disease, from contaminated air conditioners, humidifiers, water systems

Tuberculosis, from droplet contact

Gonorrhea, sexual contact

Listeriosis, dairy products, ground meats, poultry

Meningitides, respiratory droplets

Ricketts, bite of infected wood or dog tick

*Salmonella*, food contaminated by animals

*Staphylococcus*, entering through a wound, through the vagina

### New Antibiotic Discovered

A recent newspaper article announced a new drug has been found in New England dirt. Scientists have discovered an antibiotic capable of fighting infections that kill hundreds of thousands of people each year; it is called teixobactin. It has been proved in rats and other animals—all have been able to overcome antibiotic-resistant staphylococci. This may prove to be a winner against this disease and others that have developed immunity to our present antibiotics.

It has been found that most cancer is due to random changes in DNA. It has been shown that most cancers have been caused by random changes when the DNA is doing its normal routine of splitting and a fault occurs. This is new, and much more investigation into this must be done to completely understand the mechanism and the steps to take and prevent this occurrence.

# What Today's World Presents for Life and Improvement

Today's world is quite different than was discussed about the seventeenth through the twentieth centuries. We still benefit from what happened during those times and man's learning curve on existence. We have entered the twenty-first century, with many new wonders that will help man live longer and better. I will cover what I believe are major happenings, and I would imagine the readers have their own list of "goodies."

I believe you will appreciate the following discussion of areas that will improve life and extend life. They are real, and there are probably many more to come—including what stem cells bring to the party, as generally discussed in the DNA section of this book. The last chapters of this book cover stem cells as the future means of health improvement.

## Cancer

Cancer was not discussed prior to this. This is because cancer is not a contagious disease as are those that were discussed. However, cancer is the second most dominant killer of man after heart attacks, and the percentage keeps rising.

Because the average age of the world's population is increasing, there are more and more people living over sixty-five, and this number keeps increasing. The number of people living over sixty-five is mainly due to the areas previously discussed about actions taken to rid the world of certain causes of early death. Probably the one major reason relates to the cleanliness being employed by people at all ages and improved conditions in hospitals and operating rooms.

As the number of people living to older ages increases, we find ourselves with several new medical problems. We get past the old reasons for dying, and our bodies begin to fail us in other ways; cancer falls into this kind of situation. There are many parts of our body that become a little worn, and this leaves these parts more and more prone to cancer. Areas that fall into this category include the lungs, where it has been proved that most lung cancer is due to smoking cigarettes. It is a time function that progresses as time goes on and the person's lungs become more contaminated with the smoke residue left in the lungs. Lung cancer doesn't hit young people; it hits those that are continuing to use the cigarettes year after year.

Man's prostate cancer doesn't occur in many young people. Prostate cancer begins to peak in the fifties and at older ages. This is probably based on statistics; that is, the more the penis is used it may eventually cause a problem.

Woman's breast cancer is not normally found in young women and in fact is normally found in women of ages over forty. It is recommended by the medical industry that a woman should have a mammogram beginning at age forty or fifty, depending on who is making the analysis. But for sure every woman should have a mammogram every year after the age of fifty. Data indicate that in most cases the cancer starts after marriage and specifically after the woman has had children. If found early as a lump, it is being treated with much success.

Women's female organs are viewed in a slightly different way. Present-day recommendations are that young women in their late teens should receive shots of a new medication that has been developed over the past several years that eliminates these drastic problems. Young women that used to have any of these problems were flirting with death that can now be eliminated.

Colon cancer is also one of the cancers that appear in later stages of life. It is recommended that men and women have a colonoscopy at the age of forty and every ten years after that. Here is a cancer that when caught through an early colonoscopy has a high degree of success in being eliminated. In fact, this cancer can be caught before it starts with the colonoscopy. Small growths can be removed during the colonoscopy and eliminate the problem before it starts.

Liver cancer can be initiated by the continuous flow of high cholesterol through this organ. Today's development of medication to reduce cholesterol is an important action that can be taken to reduce the cholesterol to levels that are safe. All people should have their cholesterol checked to determine whether statin drugs should be taken, and this should be a yearly check. In many cases the liver is hit with high alcohol intake, and this eventually can cause cirrhosis of the liver. The drinking catches up with you at around fifty years of age, and it is a death threat for many.

Pancreatic cancer is the toughest of all the cancers to treat successfully. It is really not known why this cancer is initiated and when. It is usually in middle age, and any pains in the back should be checked by a doctor as soon as possible. Early diagnosis of this disease has some success.

Brain problems normally occur later in life. Brain issues follow the same routines as those used to prevent heart attacks. Keep your blood pressure under control, keep your cholesterol under control, and take a baby aspirin each day to keep your blood vessels unclogged. Blood clots that occur in the vessels leading to the brain result in reduced oxygen reaching the brain and cause an attack that normally results in some parts of the body being affected permanently. In a worse case the blood clots cause a hemorrhage in the brain and sudden death. Keep monitoring your blood pressure and your cholesterol, and take medications recommended by your doctor for control of these areas. It is also recommended that one eats foods that don't result in Trans fats and other fats that can cause the buildup on the inside of the blood vessels.

Significant advances have been made in overcoming these cancers if they are found early enough. In addition, the causes for the problems in these areas have been found and actions have been taken to reduce the causes. The one that I am most familiar with is lung cancer. My wife passed away from lung cancer almost five years ago. She had smoked cigarettes since she was sixteen and wasn't able to kick the habit. It is now a well-known fact that smoking cigarettes is the main cause of lung cancer. The United States has seen a big drop in lung cancer due to the decrease in men and women smoking cigarettes. Lung cancer has dropped over 30 percent since 1995 for men and over 10 percent in women over the past decade. The biggest factor was the reduction in tobacco use by men first, and then women began stopping their habit, which had been started later than for men. In addition to the tobacco reduction, the screening for the problem has increased. Where lungs were not screened very often except for obvious problems, the lungs are now checked during a standard overall check that many people have done every two or three years. This can catch the early signs, and there are now medical methods for overcoming lung cancer that is caught early. Scanning for many of the other potential areas has increased dramatically over the past decade. Insurance companies cover the cost of many of these scans, since the cost to them is less than if the person gets the given cancer—which results in costs that are much higher for them to cover.

Cancer care has become far more personalized, customized right down to the DNA in the individual tumor, according to Shayma M. Kazmi, MD RPh—Cancer Treatment Centers of America. We can now fight cancer not just by attacking cancer cells, but by reading the DNA contained in the genes of those cells to discover possible new treatment options.

*Lung cancer* is also being reduced by early examinations. Previously the lungs were not part of a young person's standard examination, but this has changed. More and more doctors are including examination of the lungs as part of the routine examination. This added step has found problems early, and steps are taken to remove early signs. People should have their lungs checked at least once every five years.

## Breast Cancer

Breast cancer is on the top of the list of what women get hit with. This was the major cause of death for women—and it's a shame, since when it is found early there is a cure. When it is found early, there is a 98 percent cure rate; even if it is not found early enough, women can have one or both breasts removed, and this in most cases prevents death. Major scanning using mammograms began about two decades ago, and this has had a major impact on reducing the number of deaths because of breast cancer. Deaths from breast cancer have dropped more than 30 percent over the past twenty years. The reduction is due to several actions:

1.  Find the problem early through mammograms or MRIs and new methods being found.
2.  If it is found early, radiation can eliminate the issue.
3.  If cases where the condition is a small growth, a selective surgery will eliminate it.
4.  In the worst case, the breast or breasts may be removed. Imitation breasts can be used to give the woman the shape she wants.
5.  In cases where the woman's mother or sister or another blood relative has had the problem and died or had the breasts removed, this gives the woman fair warning and she may make decisions in her case. Tests to determine if the woman has a certain cell condition that was also on the blood relative gives the woman the alternative to have her breasts removed without even showing breast cancer at the time.

## The New Mammogram

About 40 percent of women have dense breasts, but 95 percent of them don't know it. Why does this matter? Studies have shown that women with dense breasts are more likely to develop breast cancer. Small tumors that are readily apparent on mammograms of normal breasts are harder to spot in dense breast tissue. You can't see or feel breast density—it shows up only on mammograms. [16] In twenty-one states, the law now requires women to be told when they receive their mammograms whether they have dense breasts. (Legislation is pending elsewhere.)

Recently, Angelina Jolie brought breast cancer to the forefront with an operation called a double mastectomy, where she had both of her breasts removed. She made this decision for several reasons:

1. They found a gene BRCA1 in her medical analysis, which results in an 80 percent chance of developing breast cancer.
2. Her mother had died of cancer at the age of forty-nine after she had shown the BRCA1 gene in her system.
3. She had other family members die of cancer.

Recently she had her ovaries removed since the gene also indicates a high chance of ovarian cancer of people showing this gene.

I bring her case up because I know that many readers know her, as she is quite famous, and they couldn't believe that someone that looked as healthy as she does would have any problems. The message here: women should get a check of their genes to see if this bad actor is in their system and take actions early. (17)

There are several symptoms of ovarian cancer, such as urinating frequently, burning pain when urinating, bloating with frequent feeling of being full, and being tired. There are other more direct symptoms related to a woman's sex life. They may have back pain during sex and have unusual menstrual periods. Any of these being experienced often should result in going to the doctor and having a thorough examination, including the gene check.

## Colon Cancer

Cancer of the colon is almost completely eliminated if a person begins having a colonoscopy at the age of forty and has one every five years. Medical groups are stating that having a colonoscopy after fifty years of age and every five years after that would practically eliminate this disease, which used to be a terrible cause of death just forty years ago. During the colonoscopy small growths can be taken off the colon, and these could have eventually developed into colon cancer. Colon cancer is avoidable if checks are done early with the colonoscopy.

Colon cancer is diagnosed in about 135,000 Americans each year, and about 52,000 Americans die of colon cancer each year. For nonsmokers, it's the top cause of cancer death. An unfortunate fact behind this statistic is that about a third of American adults aren't up-to-date on screening tests for colon cancer, which may include colonoscopy or other screening tests at recommended intervals. If everyone were up-to-date, it's estimated that 60 percent of colon cancer deaths could be avoided.(18) However, the number of adults who are current on colon cancer screening is on the rise—and incidences of colon cancer and death due to colon cancer have been in decline.

### *Prostate Cancer*

Prostate cancer was one of the major causes for death in men above fifty. Here again is a cancer that can be almost eliminated if early tests are made; and the tests are easy to take. If a person doesn't take the tests and they were prone to having this cancer there is still medical approaches that can save them once the Prostate Cancer becomes a real fact. There are radiation methods and other methods for stopping this cancer from spreading to other parts of the body and causing an early death. I will mention again that every man should have tests done early in life and save a life. If one finds they have prostate cancer after the age of 70 it is usually left alone since Prostate cancer spreads rather slowly and the person will probably die of some other medical problem before the Prostate cancer kills him.

### *Cervical Cancer*

There are several areas of the woman's female organs that contract cancer that results in death. I have covered ovarian cancer (19) and there is another women's cancer to be covered: cervical cancer. This is a cancer that women didn't worry about until about twenty years ago when reports kept showing up on women dying of cervical cancer. Here is a cancer that if not treated results in death in most women. Recently a vaccine was found that kept women free of cervical cancer. The news was passed around that all women in their teens and older should be checked and get this shot, and it will prevent this cancer. It is expected that each year the number of women receiving this medication will increase; this will be a major factor in reducing this cancer, just as it has in other cancers that have been treated over the past decade. It took a significant amount of investigation over the years to find this vaccine, and now it takes actions by each young and older woman to have this vaccine.

### Pancreatic Cancer

Pancreatic cancer is the "gold standard" where there has been very little improvement in reducing the death rate. It is called the "gold standard" since the medical world feels if they can find a cure for pancreatic cancer that they will be able to find a cure for all cancers. Significant time has been spent trying to determine tests that can be done to find this cancer early in its establishment—and to take steps to eliminate it. There is no general screening that has been established that I know of or have read about. My twin brother passed away of pancreatic cancer several years ago. When they found it, they said he had six months to live, and he asked if there were any medical approaches to overcoming the cancer. They told him they could do certain things and he would live nine months. He told them that what he would go through by taking these was worse than dying in six months. He told them he would rather go forward and when the pain got so bad that he couldn't stand it that he would take morphine for the pain. Turns out he lived eleven months from the date of the finding and took morphine to reduce the pain over the last several months. Of course, this experience with my twin brother got me reading about the pancreas and the various possible causes and possible cures of pancreatic cancer if it is caught early.

Warning signs for pancreatic cancer include pain in the back that seems constant even while one is resting or sleeping. Anyone having these types of pain in their back should have a cancer check for this disease. In my brother's case the thought it was his gall bladder, and they removed his gall bladder. The pain got worse, and they thought they might have torn something in his liver while doing the operation. They went in and did some things to his liver, but it didn't help. Finally, after almost a year of pain they went in and found the pancreatic cancer.

Recently the first artificial pancreas was attached to an Australian boy. It is a small pump that senses a drop in glucose levels and automatically turns off the delivery of insulin, preventing a hypoglycemic attack. (20) There have been several advances toward determining possible cures for those affected. This could be a significant step in reducing diabetes as well. This all depends on the success long term of this procedure.

### There are other cancers

There are other cancers, some of which I have mentioned, but the ones I have listed here are the ones that affect the greatest numbers of people. The medical world continues to find screening procedures for all the other less prevalent cancers. Their great hope is to find something that is common to all the cancers and find out how to rid the body of this problem. Perhaps the work on DNA-caused issues will solve the total problem, especially for pancreatic cancer. There has been considerable work on analyzing the DNA and stem cells of those with cancers to determine if stem cells in the DNA look different in cancer growths. There have been considerable findings on how these relate to the cancer problems, and the bio scientists are looking for a way of using stem cell approaches to solve cancer.

### DNA—Relation to Cancers

A recent article in the newspaper by Jeanne Whalen discussed cancer that could be caused by stem cell division (I haven't covered stem cells yet in the book. It is described in the last section of this book. It represents the future possible cures for various diseases.). New research concludes that the majority of our risk across cancer types is due to a new observed source of cancer due to stem cells when they divide. I previously discussed how normal cells of the body divide, and the same techniques are followed by stem cells under normal conditions. A recent analysis was published in the journal *Science*, and it states that genetic mutations that randomly crop up as our stem cells divide are "the major contributors to cancer overall; often more important than either hereditary or external environmental factors."

The researchers, from the Johns Hopkins University School of Medicine, in Baltimore, analyzed published scientific papers and the rate of stem cell division among thirty-one tissue types, except for breast and prostate tissue—which was excluded from the analysis. They compared the total number of lifetime stem cell divisions in each tissue against a person's lifetime risk of developing cancer in that tissue. This was done on US tissues, and the results were rewarding and give them cause to continue pursuing this method.

The correlation between these parameters suggests that two-thirds of the difference in cancer risk among various tissue types can be blamed on random, or "stochastic," mutations in DNA occurring during stem cell division, and only one-third on hereditary or environmental factors such as smoking. "Thus, the stochastic effects of DNA replication appear to be the major contributor to cancer in humans."

These results suggest further review of the actions of the division of stem cells during DNA division. If the reason is found, it would have phenomenal effects on cancer in the world as we know it today.

### And Now Comes a Disease to Kill a Disease

Yes, I was shocked when I watched *60 Minutes* on TV the other day. It discussed how doctors from Duke University developed a technique of inserting a polio virus in a cancerous brain tumor to overcome brain cancer.

The discussion was about a woman who had brain cancer and had had all the known treatments at the time, and they all failed. It was estimated that she had three months to live when it was suggested she try a new approach developed by several doctors from Duke

University. The approach consisted of applying polio virus directly on the cancerous tumor.

The key to this approach concerns the fact that the body's immune system cannot attack a cancerous tumor since the outer shell of the tumor is too tough for the immune system to get inside and begin its work. The doctors at Duke take polio virus and strip it of an ingredient that causes one to be affected with polio; then they add an ingredient that keeps the virus active. The key after this is to be able to direct the polio virus exactly onto the tumor.

The Duke team has select equipment that allows them to hit the target exactly where they want to hit it.

In this particular case the woman agreed to have them try this approach, since she felt she had nothing to lose; and, if nothing else, it would give the doctors active information about the capability of their approach.

The doctors succeeded in placing the polio virus directly on the tumor. The woman was sent home, and she was checked with an MRI about once a week to see what was resulting. For the first few months they were disappointed since the tumor appeared to be increasing in size. Further review after four months showed them it was not the cancer tumor that was enlarging but the major effect of the immune system attacking the tumor. The key to the operation was to have the polio virus attack the tumor and break through the tough outer shell while trying to cause an infection. Once the polio virus broke through the shell, the immune system was able to begin its wonderful work.

This operation was done in 2012, and here we are three years later and the woman has no signs of brain cancer. One other person was done in the past couple of years, and he shows no signs of brain cancer today. I believe another operation was recently tried on a man who had lung cancer, and the results are pending.

The Duke Doctors believe this approach could work on several of the major cancers that result in death. Time will tell.

## What Do People Do If They Are Diagnosed with Cancer?

Almost every person diagnosed with cancer is concerned about what to do next. There is a fear to go beyond and take steps to either cure the cancer or make it less relevant. There are now professional groups to help answer the question. There is a free evidence-based counseling program called Open to Options available nationwide. Developed by the Cancer Support Community (CSC), a nonprofit group based in Washington, DC, the program matches cancer patients with paid professional counselors throughout the country. They are specially trained to help patients better communicate with their doctors by formulating questions about their treatment options during that difficult period between diagnosis and treatment. Patients can use the CSC website, CancerSupportCommmunity.org, to start their communication process. (93)

### Potential Warnings of Cancer

*There are everyday things to watch out for:*

*A persistent cough and sore throat*

*Changes in one's daily bowel movements*

*Unknown bleeding such as blood in the urine*

*Growth of a mole or a change of its shape*

*Bloating on a continuous basis*

*Daily heartburn*

*Ongoing depression*

*Any one of these is probably a reason to see a doctor to find the reason.*

## Today's HIV Actions

An estimated 35 million people presently have HIV or AIDS, and 1.5 million died from an AIDS-related illness in 2013 according to WHO.

A recent article in the newspapers relates to the search for a permanent alternative to HIV drugs. The article relates to the fact that present methods on HIV patients keep the patients from acquiring AIDS. The present methods used for those infected with HIV require that they take a daily cocktail of pills for the rest of their lives. Antiretroviral therapy—ART—keeps the virus from replicating inside the body. This status is due to actions by the medical community over the past twenty years, fighting to keep people from moving from HIV to AIDS.

Yesterday's paper discussed a new approach to solving the AIDS problem with the use of a molecule. Scientists have engineered a molecule they believe can block infection from the HIV virus. This is a discovery that is an alternative to a vaccine and is an approach to catch the ever-evolving virus, which has eluded scientific approaches over time.

A team of scientists from Scripps Research Institute and other institutions is said to have identified a way to prevent HIV from infecting cells using an approach that resembles gene therapy or transfer rather than eliciting an immune response. This molecular approach is an approach of blocking the HIV virus (94)

HIV normally invades cells through two receptors. The new molecular protein works by blocking the points where the virus binds, leaving no point of entry. Because it attaches to both receptors rather than just one, the protein—named eCD4-IG—blocks more HIV strains than any of several powerful antibodies shown to disable the virus. The study was published by the journal *Nature*.

"It is absolutely 100 percent effective," said Michael Farzan, a professor of infectious diseases at the Scripps Research Institute in Jupiter, Florida, and the lead author of the study. "There is no question that it is by far the broadest entry inhibitor out there." The trial receptors of this approach were monkeys that had been previously been proved to be excellent receptors. Results were confirmed on the monkeys, and a program is ready to be started with people—especially those that are in poor condition and would welcome this chance to rid them of this sickness. Health officials are concerned because the pills are advertised as "the pill condom" and many people might stop using condoms; this is not recommended. This drug is produced in Foster City, California, by Gilead Sciences, a giant firm when it comes to producing many new drugs for this and other diseases.

In another broad plan by several countries, The Red Cross AIDS Research Centre, the US military, and a number of academic partners are set to launch a set of potentially significant trials. Thailand, a country hit hard by AIDS, has long been a center of research for an HIV vaccine. Recent research by Thai and US military researchers to help this effort gradually expanded to look for a cure. The aim is "to achieve long-term remission from HIV." This program is ongoing, and much is expected of it over the next few years. This program is fundamental in finding either a cure or a method that holds the HIV dormant.

A study shows that a drug used to treat HIV infection also will prevent it when taken before and after risky sex by gay men. Present recommendations are to use a condom and take the daily pills. These methods are still valid; however, the new method uses Truvada, which is a pill containing two AIDS drugs. Almost 90 percent of those taking Truvada were found to be less likely to get HIV.

### *Diabetes*

Diabetes has been around for a long time. People are born with a problem whereby the pancreas doesn't supply insulin to the body. Over the course of years methods have been found and used for supplying insulin to affected people. They take a shot of insulin each day.

As the average age of the world's population grew, a newer form of diabetes presented itself. This is called type 2 diabetes. (95) In this case the person has insulin, but as he or she grows older the insulin is inefficient in handing the sugar in the person's blood. In most cases this is due to one of several reasons:

1. As a person ages, the body becomes resistant to insulin's ability to unlock cellular gates that allow blood glucose to enter cells.
2. There has been a rise in body fat as a person gets older, especially for those that eat too much and do not exercise enough.
3. Smoking and alcohol intake at high levels contribute to this problem.
4. Today's young people eat too much and the wrong kinds of food—high saturated fat content, high trans-fat, high sugar content, processed food like cold cuts—and this results in weight gain and medical issues; meanwhile, they do not exercise enough to burn off the high food intake.
5. Increases in blood pressure due to increases in the cholesterol in the person's blood, especially the LDL portion of the cholesterol.

People with type 2 diabetes may have to take insulin in a worst-case scenario; however, this is not normally required if the person goes to a diet program and exercise and possibly a mild drug that helps the body to keep the blood sugar better regulated. It is also important to keep the blood pressure and cholesterol in control.

Type 2 diabetes can be controlled and in many cases eliminated, depending on the person with this condition. They must control their intake of foods that aggravate this condition and make sure they are controlling the blood sugar levels. They may have to take daily samples of their blood and check the sugar level on special equipment that is prescribed by their doctor. They must exercise and lose body fat and lose weight. People with this potential problem should go on their computer and read about the various foods that are recommended and the foods they shouldn't eat. Among the worst foods for this condition are white bread and any food using white flour, such as cake and cookies. Interestingly enough, dark chocolate made from cocoa without sugar is recommended, as are nuts of various kinds. This is a daily requirement, and people cannot do themselves a "favor" over the weekend or during a weak moment and eat the thing that looks so good but should be shunned.

## First treatment Approved for Diabetic Retinopathy— An Eye Issue

Diabetic retinopathy, which causes bleeding and/or abnormal blood vessel growth in the retina, is the leading cause of blindness in Americans with diabetes. Deeb Hasain, MD, has reported on the first treatment approved for diabetic retinopathy. The FDA recently approved injections of the drug Lucentis—also used to treat macular degeneration in older adults—for diabetic retinopathy in patients with *macular edema* (swelling that occurs when fluid builds up in the eye).

## Prediabetes

Prediabetes is a condition that has been increasing over the past two decades and appears to be the result of the increase of the number of people that are overweight. This condition was recognized as a potential problem several years ago, but not the extent of it. It has now become a major issue; as many as a third of the people have this condition and don't know that it exists. Many do not have symptoms and feel healthy. Prediabetes is a situation that may occur before the onset of type 2 diabetes. People should keep their blood sugar level below 100 and definitely below 126. Below 100 is satisfactory, but anything above 100 and below 126 is considered prediabetic, and the person must take actions to prevent the increase to above the 126 level. These actions are the same as if one is suffering from type 2 diabetes. Go on a diet to control the blood sugar levels and take on an exercise program. Losing weight is a sign in the right direction. Again I mention that people with this condition should stay away from white bread, products using white flour, sugar, and many of the foods containing fat.

This problem is caused by the same issues as type 2 diabetes, including overweight and eating too much of foods that can exacerbate this condition. The overweight issue has been with us for several decades, and high readings on blood sugar levels began to show up in large numbers of people. More and more people showed poor results on blood tests. It's like the poison of our latest generations due to the freer life we live and the wonderful food available ... and maybe even the availability of computers and iPhones. The daily overuse of these types of activities results in too many people sitting around and looking at their computers and iPhones rather than doing physical things in their lives. It's the sign of our times, and actions must be taken by the individuals involved. There is a list of the proper foods to eat listed in many reports and on the computers and iPhones. A person only has to establish the proper routines of eating and exercising to give him or her a good chance of not reaching type 2 diabetes.

### High Blood Sugar and One's Thinking

Long periods of time with high blood sugar can result in problems with one's heart, kidneys, eyes, and now some doctors believe, one's thinking.(23) In a pivotal 2009 study in *Diabetes Care,* researchers studied people with uncontrolled type 2 diabetes and other risks for cardiovascular disease and found a link between high blood sugar and problems with thinking and memory. There are many possible reasons for this link between blood sugar and brain function, says Dr. Goldfine. One prime suspect is vascular dementia. Over time, diabetes damages small arteries in the brain, leading to ministrokes (discussed in the section on strokes) and brain tissue death. The result is a gradual loss of mental function.

### Better Glucose Monitoring

The FDA recently approved the use of the Nova StatStrip Glucose Hospital Meter System—which quickly monitors blood sugar—for all hospitalized patients, including those who are critically ill. Accurate monitoring and blood glucose control are important for all hospital patients to reduce complications and length of stay, and to speed recovery after surgery. The system was originally approved in 2006 for monitoring outpatients enrolled in hospital diabetes control programs. (97) It was found to be valuable for inpatient daily monitoring.

## High Cholesterol

I am covering high cholesterol adjacent to this section on diabetes, but it could have been covered in the sections on strokes, or heart attacks, or high blood pressure, since the issues involve many of the same problems and cures. In fact, it has been proved that high cholesterol (especially the LDL portion) is the precondition that results in high blood pressure, which causes strokes and heart attacks. So the initial battle in most cases is with this condition.

It is important to control blood pressure. High blood pressure is normally the result of several abnormal conditions, many of which are the result of high cholesterol in the blood. Cholesterol is released from the liver and is made up of HDL (high-density lipoproteins) and LDL (low-density lipoproteins). The HDL is the good cholesterol, since it essentially scrubs the plaque off the inside surface of the blood vessels. The LDL is the culprit, since it deposits plaque on the inner surface of the blood vessels. This plaque is the beginning of a potentially huge problem. A person can have a stress test done or a heart issue checked, and it will not show up this buildup of plaque, because it may be small at the time. However, the small plaque will start to engage with the white cells flowing in the blood, and this LDL and the white cell buildup will continue to progress unless actions are taken. Eventually they may build up to a significant size relative to the cross section of the given vessel (bigger problem with small arteries with small cross sections) and will form a cap. This cap can increase in size till it ruptures. A significant portion of heart attacks occur due to a rupture where the plaque had built up. A rupture of the point where the plaque has built up causes the rupture to act like a blood clot, and this blood clot can be moved along the artery until it reaches the heart, and one will have a heart attack. In other instances the blood clot could be pushed into the brain and cause the brain to be deprived of the proper amount of oxygen, and this will result in a brain stroke. The increase of plaque causes a reduction in the cross section of the blood vessels, and this causes the pressure to increase to overcome these obstacles. The combination of high cholesterol (high LDL) and foods containing fats results in the high buildup on the inside of the blood vessels. Foods containing white flour, such as white bread and cookies; red meat with high fat content; and fat from other foods are among the culprits. More specifically, saturated fat and trans fats are the main culprits in meat and other products one eats. It is important to check the content of foods purchased in packages and cans to determine that there is a low level of saturated fat, low levels of trans fats (preferably zero), and low sugar levels. Producers of packaged foods are now required to provide information on the outside of the package as to the content of carbohydrates and calories per portion. They are also now required to state the percentage of sugar. Processed foods such as cold cuts should be avoided, since they contain saturated fats, Trans fats, and sugar. These precautions are very important for people suffering from type I diabetes, prediabetes, type 2 diabetes, heart problems, and related diabetic problems.

There are many different prescription drugs that reduce the cholesterol in the blood. These drugs are called statin drugs, and one drug might work for one person and not the other. So a person may have to go through several statin drugs until one is found to suit the person. Some people, as a result of the statin drug, suffer from muscle problems in their legs or other parts of the body, and they might have to change their statin drug to overcome the problem. Eventually one of the statin drugs will prove to be beneficial and cause little if any side effects. A new study suggests that most people who stop taking cholesterol-lowering statins because of side effects or for other reasons are able to restart the same drug or a similar one without lasting problems. The drugs are especially recommended for people with diabetes or a history of cardiovascular problems. For their study, Turchin and his colleagues reviewed medical records and doctors' notes for 108,000 people prescribed a statin at one of two Boston hospitals between 2000 and 2008. About 517,000 of them stopped statins at least temporarily during the study period. Just fewer than 19,000 people had drug-related side effects noted in their medical records, and 11,000—or 10 percent of all patients—stopped statins because of those problems. However, most people who stopped using cholesterol-lowering drugs were prescribed the same or another statin within a year—and more than 90 percent ended up staying on that medication. A person with high cholesterol will in most probabilities also be affected with high blood pressure and all the bad that this brings. There was a recent article in the papers about a new drug for fighting cholesterol. It's an expensive drug, called "The first of a powerful new class of cholesterol-lowering drugs." This article appeared in a July 22 newspaper, announcing a highly anticipated drug called Praluent. It was developed by Regeneron Pharmaceuticals Inc., and Sanofi SA provides a needed option for those that didn't get results from statin drugs. It is an expensive solution, priced at $14,600.00 a year. The approval by the U.S Food and Drug Administration is forthcoming.

It is desirable to have a cholesterol level under 200, with the LDL below 67 and the HDL above 70. Since the introduction of these medicines, there has been a reduction in people suffering from high blood pressure, and improvement in the people suffering from strokes and heart attacks. It is highly recommended for one to keep the cholesterol under control whether or not one suffers from high blood pressure. High cholesterol is an indication that one has high LDL and that plaque will be an issue. As previously mentioned, it is the plaque that results in several of the major medical problems such as high blood pressure, strokes, possible ministrokes, and other brain issues and other heart problems that don't necessarily result in a stroke or heart attack. Plaque in arteries around the heart can result in the heart beating in an abnormal manner and causing a person to have "fits" about this heartbeat issue. Many heart problems will make a person fatigued or dizzy, and it isn't until the doctor does highly magnified analysis of portions of the heart that the cause can be determined. In some cases the doctor just uses a catheter and is able to view the various areas of the heart to show the problem. Most of these problems can presently be handled by a stent being placed in the arteries that are partially blocked, and this opens each vessel to an improved flow of blood and the problem is resolved. The doctor follows up on these vessels to determine if things are in order.

One of the reasons to play close attention to the cholesterol level is that one may not have the significant problem just described, but another problem called "silent strokes." This problem is caused by disruption of blood flow to brain tissue. In some cases it is to a minor tissue that doesn't affect one like a heart attack. Because of this it is "silent" and doesn't cause the normal problems of affecting one's eyesight, speech, or walking, or causing partial paralysis of a body part. These strokes are dangerous because they are not so obvious, but they cause some effect on people, especially as they age. They may have short-term memory problems, or their personality changes. They may get angry much faster than they normally did in their life. Most people don't realize they have this problem unless it so happens they have another problem that requires an X-ray, MRI, or CT scan and the problem shows up. Continuous fatigue is one sign of this problem, and one should see a doctor to determine the cause of the fatigue.

Once people realize they are prone to "silent strokes," they need to take the same precautions that people take for type I diabetes, type 2 diabetes, strokes, high blood pressure, and high cholesterol; that is, control their diets, exercise, take statin drugs for the high cholesterol, take blood pressure medicine to reduce blood pressure, lose weight, and drink a significant amount of water and other fluids each day. It has been proved that these actions work to put a person in a much cleaner state of affairs relative to the given problem or problems.

### Low Blood Glucose—Hypoglycemia

The opposite problem can exist—low blood sugar, or hypoglycemia—in some people. Low blood sugar is as dangerous as diabetes. When the body doesn't have enough glucose to use as fuel, it results in low energy to start with. This problem occurs quite often when a person has diabetes and takes too much medication or the medication is so well accepted by the body that it is overmedicated. People with low blood sugar sometimes believe that they are exempt from diabetes, but the opposite is the case; this one has it on both ends—too little sugar or too much if one eats improper foods. Hypoglycemia can be hereditary, and this is difficult to realize, since it happens early in life and people take for granted that they have low energy—not realizing they have low blood sugar. Those that usually have high energy and suddenly lose it realize something is wrong and go to the doctor. Hypoglycemia is usually the result of eating too many simple carbohydrates, such as sugar-loaded foods and white flour (white bread). Hypoglycemia is easier to control than diabetes—people just have to watch their diet and take medicines that are available.

Hypoglycemia is not as easily diagnosed, with some people showing anxiety behavior that normally may end up with their seeing a psychiatrist. This is why a person having anxiety symptoms should see a doctor who will prescribe blood tests as an initial step. It is difficult to diagnose because the symptoms are subtle in most cases. If one's blood sugar is below 70 mg/dI, one is considered to be hypoglycemic.

One of the usual effects of hypoglycemia is fatigue, with people feeling tired or sleepy. Their lack of energy is the first indication that they have low sugar, and they have the blood checked. Other signs are nervousness, sweaty feeling, nausea, light-headedness, and other conditions that relate to low energy.

There are medications for hypoglycemia, but the key is to make sure people have a proper diet. Since people may need to eat more foods with sugar in them as part of the diet, it must be monitored, or they can begin to have type 2 diabetes from the diet. There has been good success in treating hypoglycemia to make people's lives quite tolerable.

### *Newer Add-On Drugs for Improving Blood Sugar Control*

There are many new drugs for treating blood sugar problems (high or low blood sugar). Each represents an effect that may not be right for each person, since there are so many different effects depending on the person's actual problems. The list below indicates the drugs, their advantages, and their possible side effects for each individual.

The following is an analysis/summary of various drug listings along with the mechanism of action of each. This is from a Mayo Clinic health letter. One can read the total report by addressing the proper web address.

| Drug Class | Advantages | Side effects |
|---|---|---|
| Alpha-glucosidase inhibitors Slows absorption of glucose | Although less effective at lowering glucose than are other drugs, the unique action may make it a good add-on option | Gas, bloating, diarrhea—may be reduced by taking lower doses |
| Thiazolidinedione's<br><br>Makes body tissues more sensitive to insulin | generally well tolerated by older adults;<br><br>can be taken by those with kidney disease; doesn't cause hypoglycemia | Fluid retention; may cause or worsen<br><br>heart failures; associated with increased weight, fracture risk, and bladder cancer, which often limits use |
| Meglitinides Stimulates a production of a quick burst of insulin | Less likely than sulfonylureas to cause hypoglycemia; Repaglinide can be taken by those with kidney disease | Upset stomach; hypoglycemia is still a risk |
| Dipeptidyl-peptidase-4<br><br>(DPP-4) inhibitors Stimulates insulin production | Not as effective at lowering<br><br>blood glucose as other drugs; | May increase risk of colds and headache;<br><br>may increase risk of pancreas inflammation |

| | | |
|---|---|---|
| when blood sugar rises | doesn't cause hypoglycemia if used alone; doesn't cause weight gain | |
| Sodium glucose cotransporter 2 | low risk of hypoglycemia when (SGLT-2) inhibitors taken alone. May lose weight, Dehydration. | Urinary tract and yeast infections |
| | | Causes excess blood glucose to be excreted In the urine |
| Incretin mimetics Mimics the gut hormone incretin, causing insulin release with high blood glucose | Injectable drugs Works when blood glucose is high, unlike other drugs in which insulin secretion is stimulated regardless of blood glucose levels; may decrease appetite with modest weight loss. | Nausea, which often improves with time; vomiting, loss of appetite, dizziness, constipation, and upset stomach; associated with increased risk of pancreatitis and altered kidney function |
| Amylin mimetics Mimics action of pancreas hormone amylin, slowing digestion | May cause weight loss; can help with type 1 or type 2 diabetes to avoid hypoglycemia | Vomiting, abdominal pain, diarrhea, dizziness, headache, and fatigue; adjusting insulin dose is necessary |

Type 1 diabetes is diagnosed early in life; people either produce enough insulin or they don't. Their life is continuously being attacked, and they must follow a prescribed routine established by their doctor.

Prediabetes and type 2 diabetes come along later in life, and most people don't even know they have either of them. About 60 percent of the people with prediabetes don't know it. Those that are fortunate enough to have an annual physical exam will find out with the blood test. One of the problems, however, relates to those diagnosed: they may think they can get along without doing anything about it, since they feel physically good; however, if they don't take the advice of the doctor, they will realize it is for real and needs attention on a daily basis with a diet and some good exercises.

## *Low Levels of Vitamin D Linked to Type 2 Diabetes*

A recent article in *Everyday Health* stated that it was found that vitamin D was linked to a risk of type 2 diabetes and stated that it was found even when people weren't overweight, according to researchers.

The study included almost 150 people in Spain. Their vitamin D levels were checked, as was their body mass index (BMI). They also had tests for diabetes, prediabetes, or other blood sugar (glucose) metabolism disorders.

Obese people who didn't have diabetes or related disorders had higher vitamin D levels than those with diabetes. Lean people with diabetes or related disorders were more likely to have low vitamin D levels than those without such disorders.

The results show that vitamin D levels were more closely linked to blood sugar levels than BMI. What the study wasn't able to tease out, however, was whether or not vitamin D played a role in causing diabetes or other disorders that affect the metabolism of glucose.

The findings were published recently in the Endocrine Society's *Journal of Clinical Endocrinology & Metabolism*, which can be found on one's computer by going to Firefox or other related computer programs.

Keep in mind that the lack of vitamin D can be overcome with some over-the-counter drugs, but maybe the best bet is to have a sun bath for ten minutes a day for three days a week. Do not stay in the sun any longer, or you may get sunburned. People that work out in the sun five days a week usually have brown skin, and if they suffer from diabetes, prediabetes, or type 2 diabetes, they will need a medical treatment. There is evidence that people that are brown from everyday sun have a lower incidence of prediabetes or type 2 diabetes. No studies have shown why this is the case. People that play professional tennis are in the sun almost six hours each day and don't show the problems. The same is true for soccer and baseball players, and they don't show abnormal problems with the long sun time causing them to have skin cancer.

# Foods to Not Eat—
# For Reducing Blood Pressure,
# Lowering Sugar, Improving
# Diabetes, Reducing Strokes,
# and Reducing Heart Problems

There are many foods and food types to keep from eating to control one or all of the following diseases: high blood pressure, diabetes, strokes, and heart problems. See the list below.

White bread or anything made from white flour, such as cookies

Processed meat such as cold cuts

Fried foods

Trans fats in many processed foods

Rare beef—especially when it has a high content of fat

Rare hamburgers—same comment as rare beef

Coconut oil

Almost all candies

Canned foods, processed with salt added, along with other nondesirables such as sugar, high saturated fat, trans fats, and high calorie content

Cola drinks and many other sugary drinks

Packaged foods with high sugar, high salt, saturated fats, trans fats, high calorie count, coconut oil, high sodium;- review the contents before purchasing and make sure that these contents are avoided or are very low in amount

Energy drinks—have high sugar and caffeine

### Foods to Eat

Blueberries (96)—This fruit is high on the list for people that want to help keep their sugar in control while having something sweet to eat. Besides helping to keep the blood pressure down, blueberries have been shown to boost the brain as described in *Health & Nutrition Letter.*

Foods with low sugar

Foods with high fiber content, such as avocados, many breakfast cereals, carrots, and many vegetables; also peanuts, walnuts, almonds, and other nuts

Packaged foods with no trans fats, no saturated fats (or low levels), and low sodium; check the contents.

Almost all kinds of nuts, especially almonds and walnuts

Fish—not fried

Chicken or turkey—not fried and don't eat the skins

Pork—not fried and without eating the fat

Most fruits, but some people may have to avoid grapefruit for a medical condition and the medicine they take for it

Legumes—most beans are very good, with high fiber

Brown bread—whole-grain wheat, high-fiber ones

Avocados—have high fiber content

Milk, or preferably yogurt with zero sugar, such as some Greek yogurt

Yogurt with fresh fruit on top as a dessert—especially blueberries.

Cooked oatmeal

Drink more water … and more water … and more water

## High Blood Pressure

High blood pressure (HBP) falls into the same category as prediabetes in that people don't know they have the problem and life goes on. In most cases if people don't have a regular physical exam or don't have any reason to see the doctor, they won't know that a blood pressure problem is occurring in their system. There are no symptoms that stand out. One has no pain or any anxieties, and life is fine. The problem is that if the blood pressure problem doesn't get attended to, it can cause several major illnesses, such as a stroke, a heart attack, or brain problems as previously described.

High blood pressure can cause a blood clot to be pushed to the brain and reduce the oxygen the brain receives to perform properly. In some cases the high blood pressure might cause a small vessel in the brain to rupture, and this can cause many problems, including death. Likewise, the HBP causes the heart to work harder and can result in any of several major complications with the heart. In some cases the high blood pressure can cause clots to be pushed to the lungs and result in lack of proper oxygen. So it is obvious that people should be aware of the condition of their blood pressure. This usually comes from a visit to the doctor followed by proper medication if **HBP** is observed by the doctor.

There are many medications for **HBP**, and the chances are that one will go from one medication to another till the right one or a combination is found for that given person. After finding the right one or combination, the person then has to strictly follow the daily routine of taking the proper prescribed amount every day, day in and day out.

Blood pressure is measured in several ways, but the one that is most convenient and parallels the type the doctors normally use is the one where a pressure band is placed on the arm just above the elbow on the inside of the arm. There is a measuring unit built into the band, and this unit should be placed on the spot just above the inside of the elbow so it can monitor the pressure. The pressure comes from a small rubber ball that one holds in his or her hand and begins to pump up to a pressure of 200 psi—or a little higher if need be. This pressure is monitored by a small instrument that is connected to the band on one's arm and has a gage on it that displays the pressure. Once one stops pumping, the pressure gage shows a drop in the pressure being applied. At some point the pressure inside the person's arm is higher than the pressure being applied, and the gage notes this and continues to monitor the decreasing pressure. At some point the blood pressure falls below the amount needed to sustain the monitoring level, and the system stops and gives two readings: the high blood pressure reading (systolic) and the low pressure reading (diastolic). The difference between these two readings is the pulse pressure (50 to 65 is ideal). If one's measurements happen to be 140/90, he is considered to have high blood pressure. The ideal blood pressure level is 120/80. In most cases a person with high blood pressure has a reading higher, such as 190/110, and some have readings above 200/140. Recent findings by several medical facilities after a large study showed that a person over sixty years of age could have blood pressure readings of 140 and be okay. Likewise, people over seventy or eighty could have readings as high as 159/100 and be considered stable.

Let's analyze what these reading represent. They are monitoring the pressure of the heart as it beats out blood; the high reading (systolic) is when the heart is pumping the blood, and the low reading (diastolic) is when the heart is resting between pumps. If a person has a high reading above the 140 mark, it means that the heart has to pump harder to overcome problems in the blood circulating system. This usually means the heart is pumping blood into vessels that are restricted in some way, such as having too narrow a cross section. In some very bad conditions a vessel may be blocked somewhere in the blood circulation system by a blood clot. Keep in mind that the heart is beating about every second of one's life. If it continues to be beating against restrictions, the heart can have problems due to "overworking." If the restrictions relate to a blood clot, it can be forced to stop pumping blood in that given artery or vein, and this is a real problem, usually resulting in a stroke. Separate from having heart conditions due to high blood pressure, there are other issues such as strokes, brain damage, kidney failure, and perhaps dementia. The details are in the section on strokes that follows this section.

So one can have a measuring method related to possible high blood pressure with the following guidelines:

1. Normal blood pressure should be 120/80. With these measurements there is no problem.
2. If one's blood pressure is around 140/90 at a young age, he or she is considered as having high blood pressure.
3. If one is over sixty, a pressure reading of 150/90 is considered high but acceptable and should be treated.
4. If one is over seventy, a pressure of 159/90 is considered high but acceptable and should be treated.
5. If one has a blood pressure reading of higher than 180/110, no matter his or her age, an emergency should be considered. This person's blood cells are being torn up, and he or she will have at least one of the diseases discussed.

## *White Coat Effect*

People that have blood pressure measuring equipment at home may have different measurements than those received at the doctor's office. The doctor's measurements are normally higher than those measured at home. This is called the "white coat effect." This is caused by the person receiving the measurements at the doctor's office being excited or "uptight" and their nerves causing their blood pressure readings to go up. The key is to take your measuring equipment to the doctor's office and see how it calibrates against their readings.

It is important for those taking measurements at home to perform them with certain repeatable methods. The person, after applying the measuring band around his or her arm above the elbow so that the pickup point on the band is on the inside of the arm (the inside relating to when one opens the palm of one's hand the inside of the arm is exposed and the pickup of the monitor is just above the crook of the arm by about an inch). You should then sit for five minutes with your feet flat on the floor to relax your system, and then begin to pump the rubber cup that increases the pressure. Take the monitoring level to just above 200 while your arm is at a level with your heart, and release the pump. The monitor will start to show a decreasing pressure level and eventually will stop and release the pressure; the monitor will show and record high and low readings in this relaxed condition of your body. Never take the pressure when you are excited or under pressure or have just completed a physical exercise. This relaxed measurement should compare with the doctor's unless you have a white coat effect to take into account.

Keep in mind that blood pressure medication, along with any other medications one may take, must be taken each day on a schedule and not be missed. The best way I have found to make sure I take all my medications on a strict routine basis is the following:

1. Each night I put out all the pills I am to take for twenty-four hours, including the ones I take at night.
2. Count them to make sure they are all there.

3. Take the ones that are to be taken before bed.
4. Place the rest in a small cup and place it on the kitchen table.
5. In the morning after taking the last bite of breakfast, I dump the cup of pills on the kitchen table pad.
6. I count them to make sure all of them are there (in my case for the total day).
7. Take the ones scheduled for breakfast and put the rest in the cup, which stays on the table.
8. Take the remaining pills out of the cup after eating supper and take them. All the pills are gone for the day.
9. Start all over again each night at the same time. My time is 11:00 p.m. when the late news is going to be on.

I have been using this routine for forty-nine years. It is a rigid schedule and keeps me on time for my medications.

The following is a list of blood pressure medications and their effects on the person as well as some possible side effects.

### Diuretics and Blood Pressure

Diuretics are the basic medication given for high blood pressure. Diuretics rid the body of fluids, and the fluids carry salt from the body. They are often called "water pills," since their primary action is to reduce the body of sodium through increased urination. This increased urination rids the body of extra fluids in the body, and while doing so it triggers the kidneys to excrete extra sodium. With reduced fluids in the blood, it reduces the pressure in the artery vessels of the blood system. There are several types of diuretics, and some of them result in dilation (expansion) of the blood vessels, which naturally lowers the pressure on them.

There are some concerns of what type of diuretic to take. Some diuretics result in potassium being drawn from the blood. Potassium is important for the body, since it provides an element that helps improve energy. So diuretics that draw potassium may cause a person to tire easily or cause cramps. I take Aldactone, which does not draw potassium from the body. Others are Midamar and Dyrenium.

People with marginal high blood pressure may only need a diuretic.

## Beta-Blockers versus Blood Pressure

In addition to a diuretic, the doctor may prescribe a beta-blocker. Beta-blockers reduce the heart rate, the heart's workload, and the heart's output of blood, all of which help to lower blood pressure.

Some beta-blockers are (by their common name) as follows:

Sectral, Tenormin, Kerlone, Zebeta, Cartrol, Lopressor, Toprol-XL, Corgard, Levatol, Visken, Inderal, and others.

Ziac is a combination beta-blocker/diuretic.—

There are some side effects possible with beta-blockers, depending on the individual taking them.

These side effects include insomnia, cold feet and hands, tiredness or depression, slow heartbeat, symptoms of asthma, and impotence, and some women have issues if they are pregnant and should check with the doctor.

Beta-blockers slow the heart, and there are reasons why beta-blockers are being removed from some people who are taking them for blood pressure control, but who have other medical problems that require medicines that conflict beta-blockers. (98) Doctors are shifting from beta-blockers to other drugs that are more effective while not interfering with other medicines being taken; these include ACE inhibitors, angiotensin-receptor blockers (ARBs), diuretics, and calcium channel blockers.

## ACE Inhibitors versus Blood Pressure

ACE inhibitors help the body to produce less angiotensin. This helps the body's blood vessels to relax and open up, lowering blood pressure. Angiotensin is a chemical that causes the arteries to become narrow—especially in the kidneys, but throughout the body.

Common names of ACE inhibitors include Capoten, Vasotec, Monopril, Zestril, Univasc, Aceon, Accupril, Altace, and Mavik.

Possible side effects of ACE inhibitors include skin rash, loss of taste, and chronic dry cough.

As I mentioned earlier in the book, I lost my taste for about fifteen years. Ice cream tasted like pepper, and there were other odd things, such as lemon flavor was greatly enhanced. Then I began to get my taste back, and it has been fine for the last twenty years. I believe that doctors were not aware of this loss of taste issue when I started to take an ACE inhibitor, years ago.

### *Angiotensin II Receptor Blockers versus Blood Pressure*

These drugs block angiotensin, which causes the arteries to become narrow.

Common names of these drugs are Atacand, Tegeten, Avapro, Cozaar, Micardis, and Diovan.

Some common side effects include occasional dizziness, and women shouldn't take them when pregnant.

### *Calcium Channel Blockers*

These drugs prevent calcium from entering the smooth muscle cells of the heart and arteries. This is important because calcium causes a stronger and harder contraction, which causes the blood pressure to rise.

Some common calcium channel blockers include Lotrel, Vsocor, Dilacor XR, Plendil, DynaCirc, Cardene SR, and Sular.

The most common side effects include palpitations, swollen ankles, constipation, headaches, and dizziness.

## Alpha-Blockers versus Blood Pressure

These drugs reduce the resistance of the arteries, thus reducing the pressure of blood passing through the arteries.

Common names include Cardura, Minipress, and Hytrin.

These pills sort of act in the opposite direction of the other blood pressure medicines, in that they increase the heart rate. They also can cause dizziness, and light-headedness when one stands up, due to a drop in blood pressure.

There are other blood pressure medicines, and those who want to see some of them should go to their computers or iPhones to look them up on Google or another website.

In addition to taking medications, there are certain supplements that you should check with your doctor that are probably worth taking for HBP: coenzyme Q10 (CoQ10), which reduces HBP by an average of 15/10 points; taurine, an amino acid that can lower HBP by 9/4.1 points; and lycopene, an antioxidant in tomatoes, grapefruit, and other fruits that lowers the HBP. There are also foods that keep the body weight down, and this helps to keep the HBP down.

Taking a baby aspirin each day helps by causing the arteries to expand, allowing the blood pressure to drop. Those taking an aspirin each day should take it before going to bed along with the other medications you take before bed. Aspirin taken during the day loses its strength during the day, while when it is taken at night, it uses the new tablet strength during the sleeping hours, and this is more effective.

Keep in mind the foods previously listed for keeping blood sugar down to lower prediabetes and diabetes risk. These foods are important for helping to keep blood pressure down also.

## *Strokes*

A stroke is a condition where blood flow to the brain is interrupted or partially stopped.

There are two primary strokes:

Ischemia—this is a condition where blood flow is impeded.

Hemorrhagic stroke—this is a condition where a blood vessel in the brain leaks or bursts.

The ischemic stroke is one where a blood clot located in one of the arteries causes the blood supply to be blocked or partially blocked. Normally if the blood pressure is high, it will push a clot toward the brain and essentially cut off the supply of oxygen to the brain.

An ischemic stroke usually is treated one of several ways. If the person with the stroke is rushed to the hospital and is there within ten minutes, the doctors now have a medical injection that helps overcome the effects of the stroke; treatment is mostly with no major problem to the recipient, and he can go home within a day. If one arrives at the hospital within two hours, there are medications that limit the severity of the stroke, and a person may not have to stay in the hospital. A recent article in the *San Jose Mercury News* described a new improved method developed at Stanford Hospital (Dr. Jennifer Tremmel). This method works by entering the blood vessel at the wrist of the patient instead of going through the leg. Stanford has defined this approach as "the balloon" approach. They call it this name since when the person with the stroke or heart attack arrives at the hospital; they fill a certain balloon that takes ninety minutes to deflate (used to time the maximum allowed time for the procedure to ensure good results). They expect to complete their process within 90 minutes. If they do this, the person will not have long-term effects. The latest victim that was sent to the Stanford hospital was a forty-seven-year-old worker who was having a very painful heart attack, and they completed the operation in thirty-eight minutes. He was able to go home and begin his work duties in a short time. Dr. Jennifer

Tremmel pioneered this approach, known as "trans radial access," which accesses the heart through an artery in the wrist instead of in the groin. This method obviously increases the time one has to get to the hospital over the previous ten-minute requirement.

If the patient doesn't reach the hospital within the ten-minute period, then the stroke is treated as strokes have been treated for several years. The doctor could put a catheter in the spot of the brain where the blood clot, or clots, is located and remove the problems.

If the stroke was caused by an aneurysm, the person will probably be required to have surgery. An aneurysm is a situation where there is a weak area in one or more of the blood vessels feeding the brain. This aneurysm swells up and will burst if not treated. The treatment is sort of routine for surgeons these days with the equipment they possess. There are U-shaped metal pieces for different sizes of the vessel leading to the aneurysm or to the neck of the swollen spot. The U clip is slipped over the neck of the aneurysm and essentially starves it of blood and keeps it from bursting. This procedure is called an angioplasty, and it clears the blocked artery.

### Symptoms of a Stroke

There are several warning signs of a pending stroke, and each person should take them seriously.

1. Sudden weakness or numbness in the face, arm, or leg on one side of the body
2. Abrupt loss of vision, strength, coordination, sensations in hands, and the ability to make sense of another person's speaking voice; is increasing in time
3. Sudden dimness of vision, especially in one eye
4. Sudden loss of balance and problems with walking. Dizziness causing upset stomach and vomiting, nausea, fever, hiccups, or trouble with swallowing
5. Sudden and severe headache with no other reason; may be followed by unconsciousness

## The FAST Rule

There is a general rule that people should be aware of. It is called the FAST rule. This relates to the following and is an indication of a stroke.

Facial—facial numbness or facial problems that result in one side of a person's face sagging

Arms—having problems with raising one's arm or arms

Speech—having problems speaking without slurring; usually caused by inability to using one's lips properly

Take off—take off for the hospital if any of the above occurs

There is also a recommended diet called FAST that relates to the kind of foods that one should eat to prevent HBP and strokes. Those interested should go to their computers and review the FAST diet.

As previously indicated, one of the sources of each of these problems could be related to high blood pressure. It is obvious that high pressure can move clots toward the brain and cause the ischemic type of stroke. It is also obvious that high blood pressure can cause the spot of an aneurysm to swell. All it takes is a weak spot in the blood vessel, and a high blood pressure applied to it can cause it to swell further and sometimes burst.

As previously indicated, the doctor may prescribe to the patient that he takes an aspirin on a daily basis to thin the blood and spread blood vessels to allow free blood flow and reduce the pressure in either of the two types of strokes. It is obvious that people with chronic HBP stand to risk a stroke, and this is why there is so much emphasis on having controlled blood pressure to prevent these types of issues. High blood pressure doesn't kill you, but the effects of the HBP can result in one of these two types of strokes occurring, which can kill you. Doctors usually recommend that patients with high blood pressure should exercise on a regular basis, reduce their weight, and eat a well-balanced diet that is high in potassium and low in salt. In addition, medication may be prescribed as indicated in the section above on high blood pressure.

There are other conditions that increase the possibility of one having a stroke, such as type 1 diabetes, type 2 diabetes, and even prediabetes. People with these conditions are already in a medical condition that makes them more prone to a stroke. Those that are medium to heavy smokers of cigarettes increase their chances of a stroke. Those that are heavy drinkers of alcohol are endangered; however, recent information indicates that people who are light to medium drinkers of alcohol (one or two drinks a day) can actually benefit. Recent articles have been written about the effects of alcohol on strokes, and the authors hope that those that do not abide in alcohol do not start just to lower their chances of a stroke. Another activity that increases the chances of a stroke is the use of illicit drugs, dope, or smoking of drugs.

Stroke prevention is obvious, and there has been a decrease in strokes of those that are under fifty years of age; this decrease is mainly believed to be the result of reduced smoking in the United States and more emphasis on keeping blood pressure in control. The availability of rather inexpensive equipment for monitoring blood pressure at home has helped. People can monitor their blood pressure and even note what may cause increases or decreases in their blood pressure and provide this information to the doctor.

### *Minor Ischemic Strokes.*

Many people have stroke symptoms that do not last more than a few minutes. Some of them may have experienced a minor ischemic stroke. Some people are prone to this, and it happens time and again. They could be a problem, and the doctor should be made aware of them. They may be a signal that the person has a problem that doesn't fall into the category of normal ischemic stroke. Some doctors call this a ministroke, and it seems as the average age of people keep increasing in the United States that this is seen more often. It may be that this type has always been present in the populace but people were not concerned since they were not as aware as today's people.

A recent newspaper article stated that the Boston Scientific Corp's controversial surgical device for preventing strokes has been approved for sale by the Food and Drug Administration, the company said on Friday, March 13, 2015, concluding a six-year effort to sell the Watchman device in the U.S. They indicated sales may be limited because of newer treatment options that have emerged since Watchman was first submitted in 2008. Previous approval was held back because of concerns about its safety and effectiveness. The FDA gave its approval because an alternative blood thinner causing in some cases atrial fibrillation using some types of blood thinners.

## *Heart Disease and Heart Attacks*

There are many conditions that describe heart diseases. I cannot cover them all, so I will cover the general categories that occur most frequently. Illnesses that fall under heart diseases can include those that involve the muscles of the heart, blood vessel issues involved with the heart, heart rhythm issues, and heart defects that are congenital (born with). Many of the issues I discussed about blood vessels fit into a category called heart diseases. These include the discussion on ischemic strokes, which have similar early effects and are caused by narrowed blood vessels and blocked vessels. These types are termed cardiovascular disease when they are caused by vessels in the vicinity of the heart that prevent one's heart from receiving the proper amount of blood. These diseases affect men differently than they affect women. Men are probably going through chest pains, and women may be fatigued, have shortness of breath, and be nauseated.

In either the woman or a man there are a category of symptoms such as shortness of breath, pain in the neck, chest pain, and numbness or coldness in the arms or legs due to blood vessels in those areas causing the problem. Many people believe they are having a stroke since some of the symptoms are similar. One problem that relates directly to the heart is the condition where it feels like a heavy brick is sitting on the heart area in the chest. The heart cannot feel pain, and it shows up in other parts of the body, but the heart can feel this heavy weight sitting on the chest. This is a sure sign of a heart issue. Since the heart can feel no pain, the pain shows up in the shoulders or some other place, but this heavy weight felt on the chest is its clue that it has a problem.

Heart problems, in general, start later in life. Checking of the general health of the heart normally takes place at the very first overall health check when the doctor listens to the heart. Most heart problems are found today by more complex tests. Most heart problems occur in older people when blood clots cause the heart to not receive proper oxygen, resulting in a heart attack. The blood clots prevent circulation of the required blood to the heart or around the heart. This is a health issue that can be prevented in many cases by an annual check of one's blood pressure. Today there are a multitude of new medicines that reduce blood pressure. The problem is that an individual doesn't have any clues that there is a problem. The best solution is to have the proper gear at home for checking one's blood pressure on a daily or weekly basis. Many people take a baby aspirin each day, and this results in the cross section of the blood vessels being enlarged. This helps to prevent the buildup of material on the inner surface of the vessels that would normally result in a clot. The key elements to prevent heart problems are to keep the blood pressure controlled, to keep the cholesterol controlled, and to keep active with some daily exercises.

### New Drugs that Help Prevent Heart Attacks

It has been reported that lowering the cholesterol significantly will reduce the chances of a heart attack. Recent new medicine reported by Amgen Inc. and by Sanofi SA and Regeneron Pharmaceuticals Inc. found that new drugs developed to lower cholesterol significantly have favorable effects on possible heart attacks and strokes. These drugs are known as PCSK9 inhibitors. These companies are in a race to bring the medicine to the marketplace. Up to this point statins have been the major medicines being sold to lower cholesterol and have been quite effective. This new approach works primarily on the LDL portion of the cholesterol. The problem is that statins have side effects for many people and they need a substitute. This new medicine would block a protein that interferes with the liver's ability to clear LDL. Studies to date show this new medical approach is very effective in lowering the LDL. More studies are continuing.

## *Food Issues that Can Lead to Some of the Conditions Listed Above*

There have been significant studies made over the last twenty-five years on food's effects on people's health. In general, the same diet issues that have been discussed with HBP, diabetes, and strokes also affect the heart. Too much food and weight gain are big problems. The diet that one has can affect the problem. One should stay away from trans fats, saturated fats, sugar incorporated in the food, processed food that has a high content of all of these listed here and many others, potato chips, cookies, candy, cake, pie, ice cream, and the list of desserts goes on. In addition, people must increase their physical activity level; these relate to everyday activities, including walking, running, swimming, daily gymnasium workouts, weight lifting, daily exercises, and all the activities that help to burn off the daily intake of calories. These activities are important for all of the previously mentioned medical issues, such as HBP, diabetes, high blood sugar, strokes, and heart issues.

New laws passed just recently require the manufacturer to list (on food containers) ingredients per serving (and the serving size is listed), including total trans fats, saturated fats, calories, carbohydrates, and sugar content. The various vitamins are also listed, as well as contents such as potassium. A person prone to heart problems and those who don't want heart problems must adhere to a better healthy diet and pay particular attention to the content of the foods they are buying. If you are overweight, it is the first physical sign that one of the medical issues discussed may be in your future.

## *Heart Arrhythmias*

Heart arrhythmias refer to an abnormal heartbeat—beating too fast, too slow, or irregular. The heartbeat might include any one of the following:

Irregular heartbeat that feels abnormal to the person even when he is not involved in any physical activity; one can tell

Shortness of breath; also with or without physical activity

Dizzy or light-headed even without any physical activity

Passing out in a faint usually when getting up from a sitting position

Chest feels like it has a weight on it

Slow or racing heartbeat.

### Congenital Heart Defects

Some people are born with serious heart defects, and this is usually known early in life since the doctors in hospitals keep checking for irregularities in newborn children. There is a list of irregularities that hospital personnel watch for, including the color of the baby's skin, swelling in various parts of the body, poor weight and poor weight gain, and breathing irregularities.

There are also some congenital heart defects that don't show up until later in life, especially when the growing person takes on additional physical activities.

### Heart Infections

There are three types of heart infections, which affect the heart in similar manners: pericarditis, which affects the tissue surrounding the heart; myocarditis, which affects the muscular middle layer of the wall of the heart; and endocarditis, which affects the inner membrane that separates the chambers and valves of the heart. These infections have symptoms that are similar to those listed for heart attacks, plus there may be shortness of breath, skin rashes, a persistent cough, and heart rhythm abnormalities.

# Heart Valve Issues

There are four valves in the heart that open and close to direct blood flow through the heart and eventually to the lungs or to the aortic artery, which is the main vessel leaving the heart to supply blood to the body. These valves may be injured in some way such as a car accident or being hit hard while playing football, or they may be congenital-type problems. These faults result in leaking from the heart, insufficient blood flow from the heart, and issues related to the lungs and proper breathing, and the person has some of the previously listed symptoms of the other types of heart issues.

## *What to Do*

If any of the problems listed for the various heart issues occurs, the person should immediately schedule a visit with the doctor. None of these is an issue that should be taken lightly. Medical capability for handing these heart issues has improved dramatically over the last couple of decades. Even open-heart surgery is completely different. Not long ago people had to have their chest opened down to the belly button. Now the doctors have instruments and experience to be able to make a small cut to get into the heart or surrounding areas. A catheter may be inserted in a large vessel in the leg, and dye is injected so the catheter can be tracked on a monitor screen. The catheter is directed to the heart and to where the problem or problems exist. The catheter enters a blood vessel that is causing the problem due to being too small a cross section. A stent (a small metal tube that can be expanded) is inserted in the dysfunctional blood vessel and is forced to expand, which expands the blood vessel. The expanded stent is left in this position, since it provides the proper cross section to allow the blood vessel to operate properly. The catheter is withdrawn out the leg artery. The problem with the heart in this case is eliminated. Stents are applied in various places determined to be causing a problem due to shrinkage of the cross section of a vessel due to plaque buildup or shrinkage or partial rupture. Catheters can be inserted in other arteries in the arm or leg to direct a stent and solve these problems.

## Stents

Any hospital that has the capability of doing heart surgery has the capability of doing stent insertions. This is also a way to solve some blood pressure problems and some stroke conditions. Stents are also used when a person has kidney stones removed. The stones are crushed and stents are applied that lead the chopped-up stones to the output of the penis or female discharge organ to reduce pain while passing the crushed stones.

# Vaccines

Over the past hundred or so years there have been many vaccines developed that eliminate the possibility of most people suffering from a particular disease. In fact, the name *vaccine* came from Edward Jenner finding a cure for smallpox in 1798. He found that if a person was given cowpox that it prevented the person from getting smallpox. Smallpox of a cow (which a person is immune to) is termed *Variolae vaccinae*, and from this he called it a vaccine. Since 1811 the term vaccine has been used for protective inoculations.

A vaccine is biological preparation that provides the body active acquired immunity to a particular disease. A vaccine usually contains an agent that resembles a disease-causing microorganism and is often made from a weakened or killed form of the microbe that one wishes to prevent. The miracle of the human body is its ability to retain immunity against a disease for years—and in most cases for life. Once a person is infected and the person's immune system fights the infection and overcomes it, the immune system remembers and contains the acquired antibodies to prevent reoccurrence of that disease in the future.

Vaccines have historically been the most effective means to fight and eradicate infectious diseases. Limitations to their effectiveness exist, however, mainly due to some people's immune system not responding for some particular reason. Some limitations are due to the person having factors such as diabetes, steroid use, HIV infection, or age. There may be a time scale involved, since it takes time for the vaccine to take effect. The body begins to generate the antibodies needed for protection but is slow in doing so, and in the meantime the strains of the disease may take over. Even in these cases the body may have developed enough immunity to have some positive effects, such as preventing an infection, lowering the mortality rate, and providing faster recovery. The person may have a less virulent form of the disease and recover faster. These are among the many advantages to taking a vaccine.

Vaccines have been developed for the following and the Centers for Disease Control and Prevention have recommended routine vaccination of children at an early age:

Hepatitis A

Hepatitis B

Polio

Mumps

Measles—I lost a young brother who caught the disease from me and the measles would not come out on his body—only his forehead, and this causes gas to go to the body. He was three and a half when he passed away.

Rubella

Diphtheria

Pertussis

Tetanus

HiB

Chicken pox

Rotavirus

Influenza—given yearly to handle new mutations.

Whooping cough

Meningococcal disease

Pneumonia—and a second shot for older people

A number of combination injections are now marketed that provide protection against multiple diseases. This is an approach to reduce the large number of vaccinations needed by the age of two; examples of multiple combination vaccinations are pneumococcal conjugate vaccine and MMRV vaccine.

In 2006 a vaccine was introduced against shingles, which is a disease caused by a person previously having had chicken pox at a young age. The virus of the chicken pox remains in the body, and at an elderly age it may manifest itself as the shingles virus. If you are age sixty or older, you may not remember if you had chicken pox and your parents may not be alive to ask. History shows that almost all children had chicken pox, so you should assume you did. This being the case, a person should get the Zostavax shingles vaccine. It will do no harm to you other than a spot where the shot causes the skin to be irritated. This shot reduces people's chances considerably of ever getting shingles, and if they do it is much less of a problem. If you have witnessed other people getting shingles and have seen all the pain they go through and the itchy rash and burning of the skin they suffer through, you will want to get this shot of Zostavax. Some people may be allergic to this shot and therefore should check with their doctor before taking the shot. (99)

Pregnant women are screened for rubella and the hepatitis viruses.

There are other vaccinations, such as

Cholera

Anthrax

Tuberculosis

Rabies—given to those who have been bitten by a rabid dog

Yellow fever

Cervical cancer

Meningitis type B

Polio was declared as having been eliminated in the United States in 1994, Europe in 2002, and India in 2014 as a result of the Salk vaccine.

The diseases demanding the most attention for a vaccine relates to the poor countries where financial considerations limit the number of people receiving the vaccines for malaria, tuberculosis, and HIV. Most of the good work in those countries comes from wealthy people who donate huge sums of money for the support of vaccines for these poor countries that are prone to these diseases.

## *Vaccines—Also for Grown-Ups*

There has recently been a push for more people to get their vaccine shots—including older grown-ups. There are vaccines primarily for grown-ups. These include a more powerful pneumonia shot for those over sixty-five; shots for shingles, which affects older people; and whooping cough, which has reared its ugly head again. Shots for the elderly that are being pushed include those for flu yearly, tetanus every ten years, and the newer pneumonia shots. People who have had shingles sometimes make the mistake of not worrying about getting it again, but this is a mistake. If a person had chicken pox as a youngster, the germ remains in the body and shingles is what appears at a later age. Get a shingles shot, and if it doesn't keep you from getting shingles, it will result in a much milder form.

To give one an idea of the extent of this issue, just 45 percent of adults ages fifty through sixty-four were vaccinated against the flu in the 2012–13 flu season. Likewise, fewer than 18percent have received Tdap vaccine, which provides protection for tetanus, diphtheria, and whooping cough, and only 20 percent have received the two pneumococcal shots. Shingles can cause serious problems with the eyes and may cause a painful aftereffect known as post herpetic neuralgia.

### Recent Shots for Hepatitis C

Recently a vaccine against hepatitis C was developed. It practically guarantees a person with hepatitis C will be free of the disease and its effects on the liver. The problem at this time is the cost. The charge is $1,000 a day for ninety days, or a total cost that approaches $100,000 for the program. There has been considerable pressure on the company that provides this medical miracle to lower their price so more people can be relieved of this terrible disease. A relative of mine suffered with hepatitis C for about twenty years. She went to the Kaiser Permanente hospital, and they decided she should take this pill for eight to twelve weeks, depending on her measured condition. After eight weeks she was free of hepatitis C. They will check her quarterly for a year to determine if there are any problems.

### Ebola

Ebola has just come to the attention of the world again after being dormant for years. It is appearing in large numbers in three countries in northwest Africa (Guinea, Liberia, and Sierra Leone). There have been recent tests on a vaccine developed in this country. The drug, ZMapp, contains three genetically engineered proteins designed to hone in on the deadly virus to stop the disease's progression. This drug was developed by San Diego-based Mapp Pharmaceuticals Inc. The virus is grown in tobacco plants engineered to make large quantities of the virus-blocking proteins. The United States and Liberia are working together. In addition, seven individuals returning from Africa have shown the disease, and they have been cleansed and passed tests taken about twenty days afterward. All were shown to be disease free and they will be monitored for at least a year.

The current outbreak of Ebola is the worse of twenty-four outbreaks since 1976. To date the virus has infected over twenty-four thousand people and killed more than ten thousand through March 2015. (100)

Strict regulations on travel from the three countries are employed. American doctors handling the disease in Africa who show signs of the disease are flown on private jets—one person at a time—from Africa to selected places in the United States in a controlled environment. They are then taken under controlled conditions to select hospitals. The plane is decontaminated, and three days later it can be used again. To date, all of those transported and given aid for three weeks have responded well and the disease is eliminated.

New drugs have been developed to act as a vaccine for this disease and are in evaluation as of January 2015.

Results of the various actions taken show that new cases per week have gone from several hundred a week to less than one hundred per week in Guinea, and to near zero in Liberia and Sierra Leone. (100)

## *Pneumonia*

The most effective way to prevent pneumonia is through vaccination. Until now, the CDC recommended a one-time dose of pneumococcal vaccine—which also protects against meningitis and bacteremia (a bloodstream infection)—for most healthy adults ages sixty-five and older. This year they recommended the older adults add another pneumococcal vaccination, which adds up to two shots.

Each year, about a million people in the United States end up in the hospital with pneumonia, a serious lung infection that can be caused by an array of different viruses, bacteria, and even fungi. New research suggests that older people hospitalized with pneumonia face four times their usual risk of having a heart attack or stroke or dying of heart disease in the month following the illness (101)

The effects of pneumonia may be worse than suspected. A new study (102) shows that for the thirty days following an episode of pneumonia, nearly 10 percent of six hundred patients studied had a fourfold spike in heart attack, stroke, or death due to heart disease. For years afterward, the risk remained 1.5 times higher than normal. Why? Pneumonia may cause inflammation of the heart and blood vessels. To defend against this, ask your doctor about being vaccinated for pneumonia.

Another problem with pneumonia is the results one obtains just by lying too many days on one's back. Many patients being treated in the hospital for something other than pneumonia end up suffering from pneumonia. It is felt this is due to the long time they are lying on their back in the hospital. To overcome this problem hospitals are taking steps to reduce the time one is in the hospital for any issue. Recent results show that there has been a reduction of pneumonia for those patients who are released early and are prescribed physical exercise when they go home.

### Outbreaks

There have been some recent outbreaks of vaccine-preventable diseases. (103) The totals are high for measles and whooping cough for 2015.

Measles—122,443 cases

Whooping cough—31,404 cases

Measles had been declared "eliminated" in the United States fifteen years ago, but over one hundred people developed it through February 2015 for his year alone.

The highest number of measles cases has been in Asia (103,658 cases) and Africa (12,016 cases).

The greatest numbers of whooping cough cases have been in Europe (15,564 cases), North America (14,361 cases), Australia (7,491 cases), and South America (7571 cases).

China is the worst for measles, with 35,677 cases, and The Philippines had 57,564 cases of measles. The Netherlands had 12,868 cases of whooping cough; and California had 11,500 cases of whooping cough as of March 1, 2015.

There have been recent outbreaks of several diseases such as measles, polio, whooping cough, and rubella. Whooping cough showed up in 11,500 cases during 2014, killing four babies while hospitalizing many. This was the worst whooping cough outbreak in seventy years. (When I was a young boy in the late 1930s and 1940s, there were many children with whooping cough.)

### Why the Outbreaks?

Outbreaks can be attributed to four main things:

1. Lack of taking the proper vaccines. People are either being negligent with their children's vaccine schedules, or they believe they cause some side effects—which have not proved to be true. In some poor countries they didn't finance the issues properly.
2. Being negligent in their everyday practices of preventing the spread of these diseases. Keep in mind that bacteria-type diseases can remain in a dormant stage for years until someone touches them and carries the disease. Present-day practices are to wash the hands with soap and water after being away from home and using hands for doing everyday practices. They should wash the hands with soap and water for an extended period of time—several minutes at least. For viral diseases that are short-lived, one should try to stay away from crowds—especially when an outbreak is present. Viral diseases are airborne or are on a victim, and one can catch the problem from a person sneezing or just breathing the air in a crowded place like a hockey game or basketball game … or like in Disneyland, where large crowds are running around and breathing hard.
3. Opposition to vaccination. There are people that are opposed to vaccination. Some think it causes side effects. Some have religious beliefs that are against vaccination.

It's amazing that these types of diseases, which have been under good control for years, have popped up at this stage when medicine is abundant. But it only takes one of the three points listed above to have a major outbreak.

The germiest public places are the places where touch is prevalent:

Anywhere where the hands are used, such as coffee shops where cups and the hands are not washed as a regular practice

Restrooms—where the hands touch many things, and many people don't wash their hands

Supermarket checkout conveyor belts, due to leakage from foods carrying dangerous bacteria

ATM machines, where there are many hands and money carrying bacteria and no means of cleaning ones hands; you might use vinyl gloves or carry bacteria washes

At work where the candy and coffee machines are located

Borrowing a person's mobile phone

Sex with a contaminated person

Restaurants—the tables, the toilets, the water jugs, the common coffee jugs, etc.

Money—people should wash their hands after handling money from anyplace

And you can name other places

## *Summary of Medical Status*

It is obvious that we have come a long way since the fourteenth century. The combination of advances provided by individual doctors has been reviewed. Likewise, there have been many advances provided with the advent of vaccines used in the world and a better understanding of the various medical problems and solutions. In parallel with all these advances, there have been an enormous amount and types of equipment developed that help in the battles against diseases of all types. There has been a fantastic understanding of the micro world through unique equipment developed for viewing the culprits and for probing and maneuvering the various culprits. Improved communication through written work or through the computer or mobile phones has transferred breakthroughs and problem areas across the world. Government programs have been initiated to provide services across broad areas of the world. One of the major improvements relates to the cell phone. Since almost everyone has a cell phone with them, they can call 911 from anywhere if they have a stroke, heart attack, or any other major medical problem that occurs without warning. In some cases, patients with certain diseases that have gone through medical procedures have measurements done on a routine basis using cell phones like the iPhone. The doctors can set the system up for handling this on a routine basis.

We have won in several cases where a disease such as smallpox or polio is gone except in several remote places. Early in July 2015 Nigeria marked the first year with no new polio cases. However, we have to keep watching for its return. We have learned a considerable amount about mutations and their working methods and how our bodies are reliable in providing immunity in one way or another. A good example might be the discussion presented about a disease killing a disease: Polio virus placed directly onto a cancerous tumor attacks the tumor to try to cause polio. This results in the skin of the cancer being penetrated, allowing the person's immune system to take over and overcome the cancer. The future will tell if this procedure continues to work well and on other cancers.

But still the battle goes on. In the next section of this book I cover stem cells, which probably provide another level of potential that we don't quite have in our grasp at this time. But it is coming—and soon.

# Stem Cells and Research

And now we come to the great hope: the hope to cure many of the sicknesses that are not promiscuous-type illnesses or illnesses spread by bacteria, but are sicknesses of statistics—100 percent statistics. All of us are going to die, some at early ages as indicated in the prior sections of this book. In the developed countries the average age of death is going up, but when people become sixty or older, they start to wear down. Those cells we discussed are starting to have problems. Some start having Parkinson's disease at the age of fifty—or if not fifty, sixty or seventy. Parkinson's disease is primarily a disease of age, and as the average age level increases across the world, we have to be more concerned about things such as this. Some will die of heart problems, also starting at about the age of sixty or so. Some will die of hepatitis, at almost any age. Some will die of liver failure, starting at around sixty years of age. Some will die of kidney failure, usually at the upper ages. Some become crippled for life at any age due to accidents or other precocious events. The list goes on. Most people would like to live to the age of ninety or so, but if one of the above gets hold of you, your chances go down rapidly. How about senility, or the advanced cases of Alzheimer's disease, where you don't know who you are and should be dead because you have become a burden to those closest to you?

When you look at the above list, you should think about how well life has treated you and be thankful for the increased longevity we now enjoy. At the start of the twentieth century, the average life span was forty-two years. It is now around seventy-eight years. That's remarkable. That's what this book is about. It's about the diseases man has met and defeated. It's about how man became educated, and how the added knowledge from his own experiences or the experiences of others has led him to the present-day wonders of man's inventiveness. Many bacterial diseases were overcome with the advent of the higher-power commercial microscopes and electron microscopes, along with antibacterial medications developed since the mid-1800s and during the first half of the twentieth century. New microscopes and other new equipment developed over the last few years have taken things a step further. Bio scientists and doctors are able to witness—in real time—many small functions in the human body and take actions in many cases that were impossible in the late twentieth century.

Our more recent battles have been against viral-type sicknesses. This story has been about the learning curve we have been on and how we have learned. Of course, we learned from the dead bodies that preceded us and the hardworking doctors, scientists, bio scientists, physicists, engineers, nurses, and many others.

When I graduated as an electrical engineer, I was very proud. I became even more proud when I developed new things that made life easier, happier, or better for mankind in some way. Later I became disenchanted. The integrated circuits I had invented and helped to make manufacturing success stories were turning out television sets, improved cars, and games for people to play. The power required for the technical achievement of an event through the use of transistors and integrated circuits was reduced, compared to the use of vacuum tubes and the many other technologies we zipped past. I was disenchanted because these were like games to me, not something that allowed people to live longer. They didn't have the connotation of better health or longer life. They were being used for fun.

One day I visited an RCA plant in Indiana. This was in the late sixties. I was trying to convince companies to stop using vacuum tubes and to use transistors and integrated circuits—they offered reduced power needs, smaller packages, and a longer life time of the electronics; there were no vacuum tubes to burn out and other advantages. After touring the plant that made television sets, I stood on a hill that overlooked the plant and talked to the plant manager. I looked out at the land and said, "You know what, I am not proud of what I do. As I look out over the land surrounding your plant and

I see bees flying around on the flowers along this hillside, I think they do more than I do for people. They bring food and color to people so they can live a healthier and stronger life. All I bring are television sets and other electronic elements that allow man to have fun, and nothing else do I add to mankind." He didn't know what I was talking about. I knew if I stopped making these things, man would not suffer one bit less, because they don't bring anything vital to man. I went away and returned to work in a couple of days. But what I meant stuck with me.

Later in life I was to be operated on for a blockage of blood flow in my carotid artery. When I entered the operating room flat on my back and was waiting for them to put me to sleep and begin the operation, I looked around at the fantastic equipment they had. Then the surgeon began to fidget with a piece of electronic equipment that had an oscilloscope that they were hooking up to me, and he couldn't get it to work properly. He called for help, and a technician in a white coat and face mask entered the operating room and looked at the hookup. He said, "Oh, I see that you are using the red cable; it's supposed to be the blue one," which he proceeded to change. I began laughing as I lay looking up from the operating table, and the doctor said, "What are you laughing about?" I said, "This reminds me of being back at work, where the same types of things happen with the electronic equipment, and it hit me as funny." He smiled and began to insert the needle into the IV drip inserted into my arm. As he was doing that I said, "You know, as I look around and see all the electronic equipment you now use to help save people's lives, I feel good about what I do. What I do provides the electronics that allow doctors to see things better through electron microscopes and hear things better through electronics, and measure things better; and perhaps best of all, equipment that helps the doctor to operate or does the operations while the doctor monitors it." And I mentioned several other things. Before he put me to sleep, I felt good about myself and what I do for people and people's lives.

Why do I mention this? How does it relate to stem cells and stem cell research? I provide the reader with my experience because I believe it could and should provide readers with better insight into how their work might someday relate to the total experience that provides a better understanding of things you are not aware or aren't familiar with. You won't know how or what your advancements might connect to some other work and allow people to solve a problem they haven't been able to solve. It may help solve the eventual use of stem cells in medicine. Remember the discussion about the microscope and how it helped scientists to see bacteria … and then they were able to find something to eliminate the bacteria. Eventually, the electron microscope came along. This system was so good it allowed the scientists to see the workings of the DNA, the amino acids, the proteins and much more. The MRI is an invention that allows one to see the internal organs by magnetically causing them to resonate; then a computer puts the pieces together, and you see a picture of your brain or some other organ. Then there was the easy-to-apply technology called "ultrasound." Using a piece of equipment that looked like a man's electric razor, the doctors could run this over various parts of the body and see what is going on inside. For example, by moving the small piece of equipment along each side of the neck, the doctors could see the movement of the blood through the carotid artery and determine the percentage of the artery that is open and free to provide oxygen to the brain. From this they can decide whether a person's artery is over 80 percent blocked and whether an operation is needed to open it properly. The fight against disease, organ failure, infection, and many other things is an easier battle when you can see what you are working with and against. So it isn't only the bio scientists and doctors that are fighting these phenomena, it's the engineers of the world as well—and probably many others that are not engineers but have innate intelligence that helps to solve the problems. They all help the average life span to increase. It's a little thing here and a little thing there that help to bring them all together in one way or another to help mankind.

The key I am presenting here is that this is not just a medical issue; it requires invention in all forms of equipment that can allow better analysis of stem cells and their applications, just as inventions have helped in the past on many medical issues. Present-day technology allows further improvements in health by using technology equipment to augment the improvements. Remember that the solution of the genome came down to computers and their speed, which allowed the genome to be resolved to the level it has been resolved. Without the computer they would have been working on the solution for decades. Today, with the speed of the computers and better knowledge, many genomes per day can be reviewed. As I mentioned in my case, people do the best they can in their chosen fields, not knowing what impact it can have on other fields of endeavor, or, in this particular case, how it could impact stem cell research and improve the life of mankind. Look at the tremendous advances in communication through computers, iPads, iPhones, faster printers, fax capability, and the list goes on. You can help. What you do may have an impact. The equipment you produce could help in many ways to reduce illnesses, or reduce the effects they have on a person. We all should strive to do the best we can in the work we produce, not knowing where it may eventually be used.

Now let's look into stem cells and what is known at this time. At this point in time there is a great feeling that more knowledge on stem cells and how they relate to our bodies and our medical weaknesses will provide the next great step in advancing life as we know it now. Medical researchers widely submit that stem cell research has the potential to dramatically alter approaches to understanding and treating diseases and to alleviating suffering. Most medical researchers anticipate being able to, in the future, use stem cell technologies derived from their research on a variety of diseases and their impairments. When one is reviewing stem cells, he or she is involved in what makes the body tick—just like knowledge on DNA does, and maybe even down to how these spare parts can influence medicine and human life.

It is important to keep in mind that a new scientific breakthrough on diseases using a new or past technology takes considerable time. Stem cells fall into this kind of category; that is, although the future looks bright for using stem cells for solving medical problems, it will take time and patience to determine how. Stem cells are such a basic form of cells in the body that having found how to produce stem cells in quantity, one has to find where they can be used—in the curing of diseases or the development of replacement parts for the body, or some other medical problem. It often takes time to see where new breakthroughs fit. It seems it takes little steps followed by additional small steps, only to find the approach doesn't work as expected ... and this is followed by new steps. Also, many times the new approach works in mice or other animals but fails when tried in human beings. It's a tough deal, but it is so exciting that people involved in medical research are excited by the possibilities and work on their approaches, for years in many cases. Many of these research people start out to prove something only to find something they weren't looking for. New information provides a better outlook on what the next step should be.

Once an approach works in a human, the next research step is to find whether it causes any side effects or is time limited. As stem cell research proceeds, there have been many avenues tried, and some show signs of possibilities and later fail. But many of the failures provide information that takes them to the next step. As I write this book, I know that stem cell theory is now being introduced in many universities in the world. This means enough is known to provide to the students and the next inventors of the world a baseline for the students interested in the future of man. This is just the first step in the wonderful developments that will come of it. This is like electronics, where in the beginning we have considerable knowledge and are able to apply it ... and then time moves on, and the more we learn the greater the impact. Solid state electronics have been around for approximately seventy years, and we are still learning and creating new products.

The previous section on normal human cells should have provided a good base for understanding stem cells and how they differ from normal cells. Stem cells have three basic characteristics that are different than the standard cells I discussed: (104)

* They are **uncommitted cells**: That is, they are not the standard cell that one finds at the fertilizing of a female egg by a male sperm. This cell contains chromosomes that are within the original cell and are a mix of the twenty-three chromosome pairs from the male and female. That first cell

is a committed cell. It cannot change. It may be different than either of the parents (and is). Likewise, as the cells replicate, they do so as duplicates of the initial cell and its inherited characteristics.

* Like a standard cell, stem cells divide like regular cells and **continue generating new cells**. Therefore, they can carry out continual replications, like a standard cell. This is a paramount requirement.

* The stem cell, and this is key, has **no identifying tag.** (They are undifferentiated.) It is believed they can be any part of the body that requires cells—whereas the cells that form in the human body soon after conception become tagged for providing functions of certain areas of the body. Stem cells are not tagged (not committed) and are in a position to be tagged later in the body to become a muscle, a heart part, a pancreatic insulin supplier, or other things not suggested at this time in its development. As an analogy, think of empty undefined tin cans. They are empty and only have the characteristics of their dimensions but nothing more. Then someone decides to use the whole bunch of them as Coca-Cola cans, and they take steps to add everything to make them a bunch of delicious Coca-Cola drinks. They have now gained a new identity. This is the same thing with stem cells. They are like the uncommitted tin cans until someone decides to commit them to being something else. They have the value of being uncommitted and being able to be used for something when they are needed. The key is for the bio scientists, doctors, and engineers around the world to participate in the derivation of how the stem cells work and where they can be used.

In some cases stem cells are related to as "spare parts," like the parts in an automobile that are not used on a routine basis. In an automobile the spare tire might be considered in this analogy. It is not used unless one of the tires on the car fails for some reason. This being the case, the spare tire is used in its place till drivers get to a place where their regular tire is repaired. It is the great hope of the medical community that many wonderful things can be brought to fruition using the uncommitted stem cell. But it is important to know there are different types of stem cells. Some types can only be used in one type of application, while there are other types that can be used for various applications. You will see this as we look at the types.

In another way of looking at stem cells, one only has to look at how we discussed a human being is introduced into the world. All the cells generated from the beginning in the mother's body are exactly the same. They look the same, they act the same, but while in the mother's body they decide to be cells for the heart, cells for the lungs, cells for legs, cells for any part of the body—but they are identical. Why can such things be identical to each other but take on different duties in the human body as they do? This is still one of the things that haven't been determined at this time. As you read on, you will realize there are adult stem cells found in each of the different parts of the body but, at least not at this time, cannot be used in other parts of the body.

It has been proved experimentally in mice and other animals that a skin stem cell can be used to become cells with other special functions, such as heart cells, lung cells, and probably many other cells in mice. In this case they would be tagged to do that special function one wants to occur. Yet it has to be proved that this can be accomplished on a routine basis in human beings—and with little, if any, side effects.

So, what do we have here? Over time we have found that stem cells have the ability to differentiate into any type of cell. They offer something in the development of medical treatments for a wide range of conditions. This is the broad view of these cells, yet many of them still, after several years and experiments, must be proved. There has been much work on the various conceived uses of the cells, but some have not come into fruition—not because they can't, but because we still haven't figured out how. Great levels of success and potential have been achieved, many of which were on a branch of stem cells called adult stem cells, which will be reviewed in a later section. There have been many treatments for physical trauma, genetic diseases, heart issues, and problems with the brain. There have been portions of success, especially in mice—enough to see the opportunity for success—and they continue worldwide.

The one thing we hope we have is the same ability found when we were able to achieve bone marrow transplants successfully using stem cells. Yes, you read that right. Stem cells from a donor's bone marrow transplant were the way certain ailments were overcome many years ago, only they weren't recognized as stem cells. It was known that if people needed a bone marrow transplant, they had to find another person with quite similar characteristics in the blood. We now know that it was a stem cell type of transaction on all those that received marrow transplants. Let's review what occurs during a bone marrow transplant.

### Bone Marrow Transplant Using Stem Cells—Hematopoietic Stem Cell Transplantation (HSCT)

Bone marrow transplant procedures have been around for over fifty-five years. The reason for bringing it to your attention in this book is to make you aware that a stem cell procedure has been in effect for this long—and it works. Many readers will understand the reason for this remark, since today there is a pro and con battle going on about stem cells. Most of it relates to conjecture about whether stem cell technology will actually be effective in curing many of the problems with organs and illnesses such as Parkinson's disease and many others. At the same time there is a battle going on about whether it is ethical to take stem cells from the embryo of a baby about to be born or what's left over in the mother before and after the birth of a new baby and use them in research. These are embryonic stem cells, and some believe they represent life and should not be used for research. They believe it is like an abortion of sorts. This is a philosophic discussion and beyond the scope of this book.

Before considering bone marrow transplants, it helps if you understand that HLA stands for human leukocyte antigens before you start reading. Also remember that antigens turn on the body's immune system. That's when our antibodies become initiated to fight the antigens. The immune system was previously discussed, and this gives one a name to remember when considering the immune system and its work.

Hematopoietic stem cell transplantation (HSCT) is the transplantation of blood stem cells derived from the bone marrow (that is, bone marrow transplantation) or blood. Stem cell transplantation is a medical procedure in the field of hematology oncology, most often performed for people with diseases of the blood, bone marrow, or certain types of cancer.

Stem cell transplantation was pioneered using bone-marrow-derived stem cells by a team at Fred Hutchinson Cancer Research Center from the 1950s through the 1970s, led by E. Donnall Thomas, whose work was later recognized with a Nobel Prize in physiology and medicine. Thomas's work showed that bone marrow cells infused intravenously could repopulate the bone marrow and produce new blood cells. His work also reduced the likelihood of patients developing a life-threatening complication called graft-versus-host disease. With the availability of the stem cell growth factors GM-CSF G-CSF, most hematopoietic stem cell transplantation procedures are now performed using stem cells collected from peripheral blood, rather than from the bone marrow. Collecting stem cells provides a bigger graft and does not require that the donor be subjected to general anesthesia to collect the graft. (92).

Hematopoietic stem cell transplants remain a risky procedure with many possible complications; it has always been reserved for patients with life-threatening diseases.

Many recipients of HSCTs are leukemia patients who would benefit from treatment with high doses of chemotherapy or total body irradiation. Other medical conditions treated with stem cell transplants include sickle-cell disease, myelodysplastic syndrome, neuroblastoma, lymphoma, Ewing's sarcoma, desmoplastic small round cell tumor Hodgkin's disease, and multiple myeloma. More recently non myeloablative, or so-called "minitransplant," procedures have been developed that require smaller doses of preparative chemo and radiation. Minitransplants remained in the experimental domain of medicine as of May 2007. (92) I don't expect the reader to understand the list I presented here. I only list it to demonstrate there are several uses for these types of transplants.

Allogeneic HSCT involves two people: one is the (healthy) donor, and one is the (patient) recipient. This is the method that was used for many years before newer approaches were used. You probably have heard of someone with leukemia who was looking for bone marrow transplant donors. They would test the potential donor and see if certain criteria were met, and if they were, then they would allow that person to donate his or her bone marrow. This worked at a very low percentage until more was found about how the body worked and before they found other methods of obtaining allogeneic HSC donors, who must have a tissue (HLA) (human leukocyte antigens) type that matches the recipient's. Matching is performed on the basis of variability at three loci of the HLA gene, and a perfect match at these loci is preferred. Even if there is a good match at these critical alleles (alleles are gene locations on a person's chromosome, similar to addresses; certain alleles are known to possess certain capabilities for controlling specific events in the body), the recipient will suffer rejection and immunosuppressive medications will be taken for life to eliminate graft-versus-host disease. Allogeneic transplant donors may be related (usually a closely HLA-matched sibling) or unrelated (donor who is not related and found to have very close degree of HLA matching). Allogeneic transplants are also performed using umbilical cord blood as the source of stem cells. It is very important for the reader to understand that those people that successfully received this bone marrow transplant can live a successful longer life, but because the body tries to reject a foreign invasion like this, the recipient must take a regular medical injection to prevent the body's actions.

### *Donor Selection To Avoid Graft-versus-Host Disease*

The donor should have the same human leukocyte antigens (HLA) as the recipient. About 25 to 30 percent of potential HSCT recipients have an HLA-identical sibling. Even so-called "perfect matches" may have mismatched minor alleles that contribute to graft-versus-host disease.

Autologous HSCT involves isolation of hematopoietic stem cells (HSC) from the patient and storage of the harvested cells in a freezer. This is the more modern approach, used since the discovery of stem cells located elsewhere in the body that could be used. (See the following section on adult stem cells.) The patient is then treated with high-dose radiation, with or without chemotherapy, in the form of total body irradiation to eradicate the patient's malignant cell population. This is at the cost of also eliminating the bone marrow stem cells, before returning the patient's own stored stem cells to his or her body. This is a tricky situation also, since the person after this radiation has a low immunity to diseases until his body has recovered its immune system. Autologous transplants have the advantage of a lower risk of graft rejection and infection. However, the recovery of immune function is quite rapid, and the patient is soon able to resume his normal body functions. The incidence of a patient experiencing graft-versus-host disease is close to none, as the donor and recipient are one and the same.

**Sources of HSCT**; Peripheral blood stem cells were the most common source of stem cells for HSCT up to eight years ago. They are collected from the blood through a process known as apheresis, but newer methods have been found that are easier and lead to less rejection. The donor's blood is withdrawn through a sterile needle in one arm and passed through a machine that removes white blood cells. The red blood cells are returned to the donor. The peripheral stem cell yield is boosted with daily subcutaneous injections of granulocyte-colony stimulating factor, which mobilizes stem cells from the donor's bone marrow into the peripheral circulation. (92) Umbilical cord blood is obtained when parents elect to harvest and store the blood from a newborn's umbilical cord after birth. (This is the same as embryonic stem cells that will be discussed, but it is done on the live newborn baby to be kept in storage for any future medical use.) Cord blood has a higher concentration of HSC than is normally found in adult blood. (Keep this in mind to tell your children, so when they have their children, they can take advantage of this step. Of course, by the time this event happens I would hope that technology has advanced to the point where on the birth of a baby, they do a fairly easy test to tell if the baby has any issues. At s more distant time from when this was written [November 27, 2007], they may know it while the baby is still in the mother and know what to do then in situ or immediately after birth. We will see.)

**Storage of HSC.** Unlike other organs, bone marrow cells can be frozen for prolonged time periods (cryopreserved) without damaging too many cells. This is necessary for autologous HSC because the cells must be harvested months in advance of the transplant treatment. In the case of allogeneic transplants, fresh HSC are preferred in order to avoid cell loss that might occur during the freezing and thawing process. Allogeneic cord blood is stored frozen at a cord blood bank because it is only obtainable at the time of childbirth. HSC may be stored for years in a cryo freezer, which typically uses liquid nitrogen because it is nontoxic and it is very cold (boiling point −196°C). It is my personal understanding that this is not a well-known procedure to "about to be" parents and therefore this is not usually a method chosen, due to ignorance. It is also my understanding that the "about to be" parents don't know enough about any deficiencies their newborn will have that would require this procedure. Hopefully, by the time of a birth in a reader's life, the medical level will have advanced to the point that this option is academic. I hope so.

After several weeks of growth in the bone marrow, expansion of HSC and their progeny is sufficient to normalize the blood cell counts and reinitiate the immune system. Donor-derived hematopoietic stem cells have been documented to populate many different organs of the recipient, including the heart, liver, and muscle—a phenomenon known as stem cell plasticity.

HSCT is associated with a fairly high mortality in the recipient (10 percent or higher), which limits its use to conditions that are themselves life-threatening. Major causes of complications are veno-occlusive disease, mucositis, infection sepsis, and graft-versus-host disease.

Keep in mind that when a person receives a bone marrow transplant that works properly, the person must receive special shots to prevent the body from rejecting these transplants since they are foreign to his or her body. The hope is to be able to eventually, on a regular basis, find a way to use stem cells to provide the bone marrow equivalent that comes from the person's body. In this way there would not be a need to have frequent shots to prevent rejection, since the cells would have come from the same source.

## *Get the Picture?*

The fact that bone marrow transplants have been around for years and have proved to be successful led bio scientists to be optimistic that we could have the same, if not better, success in the future. Experience has shown in many cases that the use of one's own stem cells (adult stem cells) eliminates the effect of the body's rejection, as can happen when there is a donor involved. (In a later part of this book I will be discussing new stem cell breakthroughs that should start making inroads on many medical problems.)

I hope this overview gives the reader a better picture of a traumatic procedure where stem cells were the only chance for life for many people suffering from what were then called irreversible diseases. Now take into account that this is a procedure established over many years, the first where stem cells were used as the cure for a sure death. This hopefully prepares the reader for the discussion I will now pursue concerning stem cell research and, more specifically, embryonic stem cell and other promising new types of stem cell research such as adult stem cell research.

You can see that bone marrow transplants began with one approach, but experience led to other approaches, some based on boundaries set by the physical limits of the recipient. This was a learning process that took time, patience, creativity, and bright minds and is still not fulfilled to their desires today. For this reason I support the push for several types of stem cell research that have shown promise. It takes a long time from promise to employment on a large-scale basis. The details are enormous when doing the research without outside issues. I believe that politics and misunderstandings by some religious groups have slowed down progress. In the case of politics, some officials felt that taking stem cells from embryonic fluid to use for doing research was like killing an eventual person. So politics kept scientists from experimenting and moving these procedures along more rapidly. The same type of pressures were provided by some religious groups that felt the same way about the use of embryonic stem cells—that these were still parts of an unborn child and shouldn't be pursued. Recently, President Obama has removed many of the restrictions previously employed, and this should find us making more rapid progress along these lines.

First, some background. Bio scientists prioritize their work on stem cells from animals and humans with embryonic stem cells and adult stem cells, each of which may have better characteristics for specific uses in the near future. It's interesting to know that we owe most of our advances to the little mouse. Their embryos have been studied for over thirty-five years, and these studies resulted in the 1998 findings of how to obtain and isolate stem cells from human embryos. This led to further laboratory research. Human embryonic stem cells were created to provide families with infertility issues some means of fertility toward having a child. This work was done using in vitro fertilization and has been practiced for years. Essentially, the procedure takes place in a bottle, so to speak. A women's egg is placed in a tube, and a man's sperm is introduced with the idea of creating a fertilized egg. There is a high probability that the egg will be fertilized, and this procedure keeps getting improved. The fertilized egg is placed in the woman to "carry the ball" from there. Now we can proceed to see what roles the use of stem cells plays in this type of situation.

### The Unique Properties of Stem Cells

As I previously mentioned, stem cells differ from other kinds of cells in the body. It is worth repeating that all stem cells—regardless of their source—have three general properties: they are capable of dividing and renewing themselves for long periods; they are unspecialized; and they can give rise to specialized cell types. First, let's review the meanings of a few terms you will find in this write-up. (104)

**Differentiation**. This is the process where the cell goes from an undefined option to a defined option. Bio scientists need the stem cell to remain undefined until they provide a definition. They want to be able to use it in an undefined state and have it change when they need it to, preferably when injected into a patient. When a cell is undefined, it means it has not been programmed, naturally or otherwise. It is like a person's head without a brain. Without a brain, there is no action/reaction to stimuli. It is like a person who is medically brain-dead, without a connection to reality or access to mobility. In this case it is a cell without a defined task and that doesn't know when or where it will have a chance to be defined.

**Proliferation.** This is the process by which the embryonic cells keep multiplying. Bio scientists would like for the cells to proliferate without differentiation so as to have many of them to work with. Stem cells are capable of dividing and renewing themselves for long periods, while remaining undifferentiated. Unlike muscle cells, blood cells, or nerve cells—which do not normally replicate themselves—stem cells may replicate many times. When cells replicate themselves many times over, it is called proliferation. A base population of stem cells that proliferates for many months in the laboratory can yield millions of cells. If the resulting cells continue to be unspecialized, like the parent stem cells, the cells are said to be capable of long-term self-renewal. This is a significant property of stem cells and sets up the base for use by bio scientists for experiments, research, or application for a projected result.

**Unspecialized;** Stem cells are unspecialized. One of the fundamental properties of a stem cell is that it does not have any tissue-specific structures that allow it to perform specialized functions. A stem cell cannot work with its neighbors to pump blood through the body (like a heart muscle cell); it cannot carry molecules of oxygen through the bloodstream (like a red blood cell); and it cannot fire signals to other cells that allow the body to move or speak (like a nerve cell). However, bio scientists want to use unspecialized stem cells and change them to specialized cells to perform the functions I just mentioned—specific functions, including heart muscle cells, blood cells, or nerve cells.

Scientists are trying to understand two fundamental aspects of stem cells that relate to long-term self-renewal: Why can embryonic stem cells proliferate for a year or more in the laboratory without differentiating, but adult stem cells cannot? This was a rather old question, but eventually bio scientists found that adult stem cells can proliferate for long periods of time. (I will be discussing this in a later section of this book.) And what are the factors in living organisms that normally regulate stem cell proliferation and self-renewal? These represent the most significant issues, since having a stem cell and putting it into some use is one thing, but having it remain vital and provide proliferation and self-renewal is fundamental for success. However, there may be special applications that bio scientists will achieve for use where they want to limit the time and turn off a function that is established.

Discovering the answers to these questions may make it possible to understand how cell proliferation is regulated during normal embryonic development or during the abnormal cell division that leads to cancer. Importantly, such information would enable scientists to grow embryonic and adult stem cells more efficiently in the laboratory. Some answers have been found in the past seventeen years, but it seems that there is still a long way to go. It would be significant if stem cells provide a look at the production of a cancer while being monitored. This would give them information they do not normally find with random cancer as it now proliferates.

The specific factors and conditions that allow stem cells to remain unspecialized are of great interest to scientists. It has taken scientists many years of trial and error to learn to grow stem cells in the laboratory without them spontaneously differentiating into specific cell types. For example, it took twenty years to learn to grow embryonic stem cells in the laboratory following the development of conditions for growing mouse stem cells. (This long time span is one of the main reasons a great deal of time and effort remain on this subject.) The use of stem cells in humans rather than in mice is still quite limited. Much still has to be learned from the experiments with the little animals prior to carrying out the same experiments on humans. The political and questionable moral issues have also held these programs back for many years, but advances in the methods have begun to move things more rapidly now. Therefore, an important area of research is understanding the signals in a mature organism that cause a stem cell population to proliferate and remain unspecialized until the cells are needed for repair of a specific tissue. Such information is critical for scientists to be able to grow large numbers of unspecialized stem cells in the laboratory for further experimentation.

### Differentiation

Stem cells can give rise to specialized cells. When unspecialized stem cells give rise to specialized cells, the process is *differentiation*. Scientists have been learning over the past seventeen years to understand the signals inside and outside cells that trigger stem cell differentiation. The internal signals are controlled by a cell's genes, which are interspersed across long strands of DNA and carry coded instructions for all the structures and functions of a cell. The external signals for cell differentiation include chemicals secreted by other cells, physical contact with neighboring cells, and certain molecules in the microenvironment. The hope is to also cause differentiation controlled by signals from an experimenter to cause a target function. Remember I mentioned that cells developed in a woman during her pregnancy are all alike, but when they form the heart they act differently than when they are in the lungs. This is key when you consider stem cells and that their actions when located in the body have to have this same capability.

Therefore, many questions about stem cell differentiation remain. For example, are the internal and external signals for cell differentiation similar for all kinds of stem cells? Can specific sets of signals be identified that promote differentiation into specific cell types? Addressing these questions is critical because the answers may lead scientists to find new ways of controlling stem cell differentiation in the laboratory, thereby growing cells or tissues that can be used for specific purposes, including cell-based therapies.

## *Embryonic Stem Cells*—As Their Name Suggests, Are Derived from Embryos

There are two types of embryonic stem cells: The first involves those cells derived from a woman's uterus. Embryonic stem cells are derived from embryos at a developmental stage before the time that implantation would normally occur in the uterus. Fertilization normally occurs in the oviduct, and during the first few days, a series of cleavage divisions occur as the embryo (presently called a Zygote) travels down the oviduct and into the uterus. (60) Each of the cells (*blastomeres*) of these cleavage-stage embryos is undifferentiated. Each of these blastomeres has the potential to give rise to any cell of the body.

In order to obtain embryonic stem cells, these cells are removed before the first differentiation event, which occurs at approximately five days of development in humans, when an outer layer of cells is committed to becoming part of the placenta. (This is an interesting fact that I had previously discussed; i.e., that in a human being the first task in the development of the baby is the development of the placenta. It is believed that this is why the human has such a large brain, due to the protection this provides in the womb.) The inner cell mass (ICM) cells have the potential to generate any cell type of the body. So if embryonic stem cells are desired, they must be taken up at this point. But after implantation, they are quickly depleted, as they differentiate to other cell types with more limited potential (in other words, they start to become different parts of the body during this time). If the ICM is removed from its normal embryonic environment and cultured under appropriate conditions, the ICM-derived cells can continue to proliferate and replicate themselves indefinitely and still maintain the developmental potential to form any cell type of the body. They essentially obtain the level of *pluripotency*. These pluripotent, ICM-derived cells are embryonic stem cells (ES). Incidentally, I mentioned that cells after the first five days would normally begin to develop the placenta. It's interesting that this would have been the first step in the normal process because many scientists believe that the human-evolved placenta is one of the characteristics that makes a human unique and may be the reason the human brain is larger and capable of higher intellect.

The second method relates to embryonic stem cells that are derived from embryos that develop from eggs that have been fertilized in an in vitro fertilization clinic and then donated for research purposes, with informed consent of the donors. These cells were fertilized in vitro for infertile couples. The female egg is fertilized by sperm donated from the husband, in most cases. Such embryos are not derived from eggs fertilized in a woman's body. In the case of in vitro fertilization, many fertilized eggs remain after the medical procedure is completed, and the resulting embryonic stem cells would be thrown away. With the present understanding of the use of embryonic stem cells for medical research, there are more donors giving their consent to the scientific community for their work. This method separates out arguments from the individuals that reject embryonic stem cells, since they are extraneous from the female body and have no chance of being a child.

The embryos from which human embryonic stem cells are derived are typically four or five days old and are a hollow microscopic ball of cells called the *blastocyst*. The blastocyst includes three structures: *trophoblast*, which is the layer of cells that surrounds the blastocyst; *blastocoel*, which is the hollow cavity inside the blastocyst; and *inner cell mass*, which is a group of approximately thirty cells at one end of the blastocoel and are the ones bio scientists select for their work.

Growing cells in the laboratory is known as cell culture. Human embryonic stem cells are isolated by transferring the inner cell mass into a plastic laboratory culture dish that contains a nutrient broth known as a culture medium. The cells divide and spread over the surface of the dish. The inner surface of the culture dish is typically coated with mouse embryonic skin cells that have been treated so they will not divide. This coating layer of cells is called the feeder layer. The reason for having the mouse cells in the bottom of the culture dish is to provide the inner cell mass cells with a sticky surface to which they can attach. Also, the feeder cells release nutrients into the culture medium. Recently, scientists have begun to devise ways of growing embryonic stem cells without the mouse feeder cells, because of the risk that viruses or other macromolecules in the mouse cells may be transmitted to the human cells. This is a significant scientific advancement. I should mention that the above methods were those I knew of late in the first decade of this century. More recent means of doing these practices are probable and should be sought by any of the readers interested in stem cell research articles that are now available.

## *Pluripotent/Embryonic Stem Cell Line*

Over the course of several days, the cells of the inner cell mass proliferate and begin to crowd the culture dish. When this occurs, they are removed gently and plated into several fresh culture dishes. The process of replating the cells is repeated many times and for many months and is called *subculturing*. Each cycle of subculturing the cells is referred to as passage. After six months or more, the original thirty cells of the inner cell mass have yielded millions of embryonic stem cells. Embryonic stem cells that have proliferated in cell culture for six or more months without differentiating are pluripotent and appear genetically normal; they are referred to as an *embryonic stem cell line*.

Once cell lines are established, or even before that stage, batches of them can be frozen and shipped to other laboratories for further culture and experimentation.

## *Testing for Embryonic Cells*

At various points during the process of generating embryonic stem cell lines, scientists test the cells to see whether they exhibit the fundamental properties that make them embryonic stem cells. This process, called *characterization*, mainly assesses their ability to continue dividing without differentiation occurring.

As yet (to my knowledge), scientists who study human embryonic stem cells have not agreed on a standard battery of tests that measure the cells' fundamental properties. Also, scientists acknowledge that many of the tests they use may not be good indicators of the cells' most important biological properties and functions. Nevertheless, laboratories that grow human embryonic stem cell lines use several kinds of tests. These tests might include the following:

* Growing and subculturing the stem cells for many months. This ensures that the cells are capable of long-term self-renewal. Scientists inspect the cultures on a routine basis through a microscope to see that the cells look healthy and remain undifferentiated.
* Using specific techniques to determine the presence of surface markers that are found only on undifferentiated cells.
* Testing for the presence of a protein called Oct-4, which undifferentiated cells typically make. Oct-4 is a transcription factor, meaning that it helps genes turn on and off at the right time, which is an important part of the processes of cell differentiation and embryonic development.
* Examining the chromosomes under a microscope to assess whether the chromosomes remain undamaged or if the number of chromosomes has changed. It does not detect genetic mutations in the cells.
* Determining whether the cells can be sub cultured after freezing, thawing, and replating.
* Testing whether the human embryonic stem cells are pluripotent by (1) allowing the cells to differentiate spontaneously in cell culture; (2) manipulating the cells so they will differentiate to form specific cell types; or (3) injecting the cells into an immunosuppressed mouse to test for the formation of a benign tumor called a *teratoma*. Teratomas typically contain a mixture of many differentiated or partly differentiated cell types—indications that the embryonic stem cells are capable of differentiating into multiple cell types.
* Probably more recent methods of which I am unaware.

As long as the embryonic stem cells in culture are grown under certain conditions, they can remain undifferentiated (unspecialized). But if cells are allowed to clump together to form embryonic bodies, they begin to differentiate spontaneously. They can form muscle cells, nerve cells, and many other cell types. Although spontaneous differentiation is a good indication that a culture of embryonic stem cells is healthy, it is not an efficient way to produce cultures of specific cell types. It does show the capability that is required if the bio scientist wants to carry this to the next level.

So, to generate cultures of specific types of differentiated cells—heart muscle cells, blood cells, or nerve cells, for example—scientists try to control the differentiation of embryonic stem cells. They change the chemical composition of the culture medium, alter the surface of the culture dish, or modify the cells by inserting specific genes. Through years of experimentation, scientists have established some basic protocols, or "recipes," for the directed differentiation of embryonic stem cells into certain specific cell types. There are probably more recent recipes that I am not aware of. Those interested should look the subject up with their computers or other means.

If scientists can reliably direct the differentiation of embryonic stem cells into specific cell types, they may be able to use the resulting differentiated cells to treat certain diseases at some point in the future. Diseases that might be treated by transplanting cells generated from human embryonic stem cells include Parkinson's disease, diabetes, traumatic spinal cord injury, Purkinje cell degeneration, Duchene muscular dystrophy, heart disease, and vision and hearing loss.

### Adult Stem Cells

Great levels of success and potential success have been proved over the past ten years for adult stem cells. An *adult stem cell* is an undifferentiated cell found among differentiated cells in a tissue or organ. (60) It can renew itself and can differentiate to yield the major specialized cell types of the tissue or organ from which it was derived. The adult stem cell was not discovered until recently (except for those for bone marrow use). There are several reasons why they took longer to recognize: One, they are not frequent in the tissue or organ. You might find one out of a million cells you inspect. Two, the main reason is the lack of pursuing this cell due to ignorance. To give you an example, if you were to take pure water from a stream and look at the cells, you may take days to find an adult stem cell, and unless you were knowledgeable on the subject you would probably not know what to do with it. The primary roles of adult stem cells in a living organism are to maintain and repair the tissue in which they are found. Some scientists now use the term *somatic stem cell* instead of adult stem cell. While the origins of embryonic stem cells, which are defined by their origin (inner cell mass of blastocyst), are well known, the origin of adult stem cells in mature tissues is unknown. (This may not be a fact today.)

Scientists became familiar with the adult embryonic stem cell, and as their knowledge grew, they began to look throughout the body for some signs of a cell of this nature. It is now known that they can be found in almost every cell location of the body. One had to look hard and know what to look for and how to look. They are minor in number compared to the normal differentiated cells. The discovery of adult stem cells reminds me of an analogous situation that I wrote about in the early parts of this book related to heavy water. Heavy water is found in every water source, but it is hard to find unless one knows what to look for. There is approximately one heavy water molecule for every thousand or so normal molecules. Once you know what to look for, they are easy to find. Evidently, adult stem cells exist in every part of the body, and they probably look slightly different to the viewer in the different parts of the body. But they are there, and very recent experience is finding them readily available. This may be the next major impact on stem cell research—in fact, it may be here already. More of the recent articles on stem cells contain work on adult stem cells. It was originally thought that the biggest advantage for an adult stem cell related to how it can be used for the given function it was found in. For example, if one found an adult stem cell in a muscle, the scientists' work usually was directed toward finding how this cell could be used to solve muscle problems.

Much has been learned, and in 2009 the FDA approved the first human clinical trials using embryonic stem cells. Embryonic stem cells are able to be all the cell types of the body, but adult stem cells have been limited to tissues of their origin, such as muscle use or skin tissue use. Scientists are hopeful that work on adult stem cells for given functions will be less difficult than using embryonic cells for all functions. In addition, it is believed that progress on the use for the specific functions can provide information on how to use the embryonic cells to work in that same location. Some stem cell researchers are working to develop techniques of isolating stem cells that are as potent as embryonic stem cells and don't require a human embryo. One example that was being worked on by Harvard researchers, headed up by Kevin Eggan, was attempting to transfer the nucleus of a somatic cell into an existing embryonic stem cell, thus creating a new stem cell line (they have probably completed their work on this by now).

Another study, published in August 2006, also indicates that differentiated cells can be reprogrammed to an embryonic-like state by introducing four specific factors, resulting in induced pluripotent stem cells.

Researchers at Advanced Cell Technology, led by Robert Lanza, reported the successful derivation of a stem cell line using a process similar to preimplantation genetic diagnosis, in which a single blastomere is extracted from a blastocyst. Lanza announced that his team had succeeded in producing three new stem cell lines without destroying the parent embryos. Anthony Atala of Wake Forest University says that the fluid surrounding the fetus has been found to contain stem cells that, when utilized correctly, "can be differentiated towards cell types such as fat, bone, muscle, blood vessel, nerve and liver cells."

### *Plasticity of Adult Stem Cells*

Adult stem cells are cells removed from an adult's tissue. They typically generate the cell type of the tissue in which they reside. A blood-forming adult stem cell in the bone marrow, for example, normally gives rise to the many types of blood cells, such as red blood cells, white blood cells, and platelets. Until recently, it had been thought that a blood-forming cell in the bone marrow—called a hematopoietic stem cell (which we have discussed)—could not give rise to the cells of a very different tissue, such as nerve cells in the brain. However, a number of experiments over the last several years have raised the possibility that stem cells from one tissue may be able to give rise to cell types of a completely different tissue type, a phenomenon known as *plasticity*. Examples of plasticity include blood cells becoming neurons, liver cells that can be made to produce insulin and hematopoietic stem cells that can develop into heart muscle. Therefore, exploring the possibility of using adult stem cells for cell-based therapies has become a very active area of investigation by researchers. This research is not subject to the politics that affect embryonic cell research. No unborn babies are lost when researching adult stem cells for high plasticity.

Research on adult stem cells has recently generated a great deal of excitement. Scientists have found adult stem cells in many more tissues than they once thought possible. This finding has led scientists to ask whether adult stem cells could be used for transplants. In fact, adult blood-forming stem cells from bone marrow have been used in transplants for forty years. Certain kinds of adult stem cells seem to have the ability to differentiate into a number of various cell types, given the right conditions. If differentiation of adult stem cells can be controlled in the laboratory, these cells may become the basis of therapies for many serious common diseases.

## Some History on Adult Stem Cells

The history of research on adult stem cells began about fifty years ago. In the 1960s, researchers discovered that the bone marrow contains at least two kinds of stem cells. One population, hematopoietic stem cells, forms all the types of blood cells in the body. A second population, called bone marrow stromal cells, was discovered a few years later. Stromal cells are a mixed cell population that generates bone, cartilage, fat, and fibrous connective tissue.

Also in the 1960s, scientists who were studying rats discovered two regions of the brain that contained dividing cells, which become nerve cells. Despite these reports, most scientists believed that new nerve cells could not be generated in the adult brain. It was not until the 1990s that scientists agreed that the adult brain does contain stem cells that are able to generate the brain's three major cell types:

* astrocytes, which are no neuronal cells
* oligodendrocytes, which are no neuronal cells
* neurons, or nerve cells

Adult stem cells have been identified in many organs and tissues. One important point to understand about adult stem cells is that there are a very small number of adult stem cells in each tissue. Stem cells are thought to reside in a specific area of each tissue, where they may remain quiescent (no dividing) for many years until they are activated by disease or tissue injury. The adult tissues reported to contain stem cells include the brain, bone marrow, peripheral blood, blood vessels, skeletal muscle, skin, and liver. Here's an analogy: the small numbers of stem cells located in the various parts of the body are like spare car parts. Automotive dealers carry spare parts for their cars because they fail at times and need to be replaced, or the car doesn't move. Maybe the small number of adult stem cells in the various parts of the body is nature's way of helping to resolve some normal failings of our bodies over the years. Maybe parts wear out. I have had an experience that is a perfect example of this.

As I discussed earlier; In 1982 I began to lose the ability to taste on the right side of my mouth, and over the next two years I lost all taste. So eating was done just to fulfill my daily requirements for food. In many cases I suffered from strange reactions to food. For example, I couldn't eat ice cream because it acted like I had placed pepper in my mouth. After I ate, my mouth had an odd feeling for a couple of hours. I started a procedure after eating that eliminated this problem. I would take Listerine and wash out my mouth by swishing the Listerine around in my mouth for thirty-five seconds and then expectorating it. After this I gargled with water to dilute the Listerine and cleanse my mouth and throat with the diluted Listerine. I would do this with water six times. Then I was finished, and my mouth didn't have the funny feeling any longer. This condition was originally believed to be due to a tumor on my brain, but they never found one. Fifteen or eighteen years later, I began to have some ability to taste returning to the right side of my mouth. Over the course of a year I could taste at about a 70 percent level. I went to the doctors, and do you know what they said in 2003? They said that some part of my brain that allowed a person to taste probably had stopped working, and over the years the body finds a way with "stem cells" (it was popular about that time to relate things of this nature to stem cells) to create a new path to the brain. They said, "Maybe that's why you can now taste." Maybe their wild guess was right. Maybe it was the spare parts syndrome. Anyhow, I have been able to taste since then, and I can eat ice cream without the pepper taste.

Scientists in many laboratories are trying to find ways to grow adult stem cells in cell culture and manipulate them to generate specific cell types so they can be used to treat injury or disease. Some examples of potential treatments include replacing the dopamine-producing cells in the brains of Parkinson's patients, developing insulin-producing cells for type I diabetes patients, and repairing damaged heart muscle following a heart attack.

### *Testing Adult Stem Cells*

Scientists do not agree on the criteria that should be used to identify and test adult stem cells. However, they often use one or more of the following methods:

(1) Labeling the cells in living tissue with molecular markers and then determining the specialized cell types they generate
(2) Removing the cells from a living animal, labeling them in cell culture, and transplanting them back into another animal to determine whether the cells repopulate their tissue of origin
(3) Isolating the cells, growing them in cell culture, and manipulating them, often by adding growth factors or introducing new genes, to determine what differentiated cells types they can become
(4) Taking a small amount of the total and allowing them to touch each other and see what the results are; this tells them what to expect from the ones that are still available
(5) Probably more recent new ways

Also, a single adult stem cell should be able to generate a line of genetically identical cells—known as a clone—which then gives rise to all the appropriate differentiated cell types of the tissue. Scientists tend to show either that a stem cell can give rise to a clone of cells in cell culture, or that a purified population of candidate stem cells can repopulate the tissue after transplant into an animal. Recently, by infecting adult stem cells with a virus that gives a unique identifier to each individual cell, scientists have been able to demonstrate that individual adult stem cell clones have the ability to repopulate injured tissues in a living animal.

### Hematopoietic and Stromal Stem Cell Differentiation

In a living animal, adult stem cells can divide for a long period and give rise to mature cell types that have the characteristic shapes and specialized structures and functions of a particular tissue. The following are examples of differentiation pathways of adult stem cells:

* Hematopoietic stem cells give rise to all the types of blood cells: red blood cells, B lymphocytes, T lymphocytes, natural killer (NK) cells, neutrophils, basophils, eosinophils, monocytes, macrophages, and platelets.
* Bone marrow stromal cells give rise to a variety of cell types: bone cells (osteocytes), cartilage cells (chondrocytes), fat cells (adipocytes), and other kinds of connective tissue cells such as those in tendons.
* Neural stem cells in the brain give rise to its three major cell types: nerve cells (neurons) and two categories of no neuronal cells—astrocytes and oligodendrocytes.
* Epithelial stem cells in the lining of the digestive tract occur in deep crypts and give rise to several cell types: absorptive cells, goblet cells, Paneth cells, and enteroendocrine cells.
* Skin stem cells occur in the basal layer of the epidermis and at the base of hair follicles. The epidermal stem cells give rise to keratinocytes, which migrate to the surface of the skin and form a protective layer. The follicular stem cells can give rise to both the hair follicle and the epidermis.

## *Plasticity of Adult Stem Cells*

Human embryonic and adult stem cells each have advantages and disadvantages regarding potential use for cell-based regenerative therapies. Of course, adult and embryonic stem cells differ in the number and type of differentiated cells types they can become; embryonic stem cells can become all cell types of the body because they are pluripotent. Adult stem cells are generally limited to differentiating into the various cell types of their tissue of origin. However, some evidence suggests that adult stem cell plasticity may exist, increasing the number of cell types a given adult stem cell can become. They can become pluripotent.

Large numbers of embryonic stem cells can be relatively easily grown in culture, while adult stem cells are rare in mature tissues, and methods for expanding their numbers in cell culture are being developed. This is an important distinction, as large numbers of cells are needed for stem cell replacement therapies.

A potential advantage of using stem cells from an adult is that the patient's own cells could be expanded in culture and then reintroduced into the patient. The use of the patient's own adult stem cells would mean that the cells would not be rejected by the immune system. This represents a significant advantage, as immune rejection is a difficult problem that can only be circumvented with immunosuppressive drugs.

Embryonic stem cells from a donor introduced into a patient could cause transplant rejection. However, whether the recipient would reject donor embryonic stem cells has not been determined in human experiments, but this has proved successful in mice. I am sure there is later data on this that the reader might know of or want to investigate.

## *Potentials for Human Stem Cells*

There are many ways in which human stem cells can be used in basic research and in clinical research. However, many technical hurdles exist between the promise of stem cells and the realization of these promises, which will only be overcome through continued intensive stem cell research. Other than the use of stem cells for bone marrow transplants, embryonic or adult stem cells have not been tried on a human as of this date (late in the first decade of this century). All experiments have been done on animals.

As I indicated earlier, stem cell technology is now being introduced to many universities in this and other countries. This places known technology related to stem cells among the bright minds of the young, and if things go as they have in the past, this is just the first step in the growth of talent and inventiveness of this technology. Bright minds come up with unique ideas that cultivate a new technology, and I see no reason why it won't promote significant advances in the next five years.

Studies of human embryonic stem cells may yield information about the complex events that occur during human development. A primary goal is to identify how undifferentiated stem cells become differentiated. Scientists know that turning genes on and off is central to this process. Some of the most serious medical conditions, such as cancer and birth defects, are due to cell division differentiation. A better understanding of the genetic and molecular controls of these processes may yield information about how such diseases arise and suggest new strategies for therapy. A significant hurdle to this use and most uses of stem cells is that scientists do not yet fully understand the signals that turn specific genes on and off to influence the differentiation of the stem cell. Further trials with mice and animals that are more complex or more like humans, such as monkeys, will be part of the learning curve that scientists must pursue to find the key means of activating this "turn on" signal.

## Human Stem Cells for Use in the Testing of Drugs

Human stem cells are currently being used to test new drugs. For example, new medications could be tested for safety on differentiated cells generated from human pluripotent cell lines. It may be possible to test these drugs by applying them to the laboratory Petri dishes where cells are grown. One could determine if there is rejection of a drug by the cells, or an allergic reaction, without applying them to a person. Other kinds of cell lines are already used in this way. Cancer cell lines, for example, are used to screen potential antitumor drugs. But the availability of pluripotent stem cells would allow drug testing in a wider range of cell types. However, to screen drugs effectively, the conditions must be identical when comparing different drugs. Therefore, scientists will have to be able to precisely control the differentiation of stem cells into the specific cell type on which drugs will be tested. "Current knowledge" of the signals controlling differentiation falls well short of being able to mimic these conditions precisely enough to consistently have identical differentiated cells for each drug being tested. I quoted "current knowledge" because there has been significant progress made over the last several months, and signals have been located for certain functions. New medications have recently been used to test for safety on differentiated cells generated from human pluripotent cell lines. As previously mentioned Cancer cell lines are used to screen potential antitumor drugs. One of the most important applications of human stem cells is the generation of cells and tissues that could be used for cell-based therapies. The need for transferrable tissues and organs is much greater than the supply available. Stem cells could improve the number available if the control of stem cell differentiation for a particular application, such as for a stroke and others, could be properly controlled.

The use of both embryonic and adult-derived stem cells for cardiac repair is an active program in several places around the world. There have been studies on patients undergoing heart surgery, and several have demonstrated that stem cells can be injected into the heart or the circulatory area to induce the formation of new capillaries. Scientists must be able to manipulate stem cells so that the proper characteristics for successful differentiation, transplantation, and engraftment are available. Improvements in these areas continue with some success.

Remember earlier information about DNA and how the mRNA carries the triplets called codons out of the nucleus? These codons, along with the anticodons, generate the amino acids that then are used to construct the proteins needed by the body. Scientists have been able to change one nucleotide in a triplet, which results in major changes in mice and other animals. The same type of path that that applied to determining the genome of man and how this allowed a better understanding of what gene affects which function will be likely followed on the stem cell learning curve. It requires continual work on the issue to develop the learning curve to discover these details about the stem cell.

Perhaps the most important potential application of human stem cells is the generation of cells and tissues that could be used for cell-based therapies. Today, donated organs and tissues are often used to replace ailing or destroyed tissue, but the need for transplantable tissues and organs far outweighs the available supply. Stem cells, directed to differentiate into specific cell types, offer the possibility of a renewable source of replacement cells and tissues to treat diseases and other conditions, including Parkinson's and Alzheimer's diseases, spinal cord injury, stroke, burns, heart disease, diabetes, osteoarthritis, and rheumatoid arthritis.

For example, it may become possible to generate healthy heart muscle cells in the laboratory and then transplant those cells into patients with chronic heart disease. Preliminary research in mice and other animals indicates that bone marrow stem cells, transplanted into a damaged heart, can generate heart muscle cells and successfully repopulate the heart tissue. Other recent studies of cell culture systems indicate that it may be possible to direct the differentiation of embryonic stem cells or adult bone marrow cells into heart muscle cells. In people who suffer from type 1 diabetes, the cells of the pancreas that normally produce insulin are destroyed by the patient's own immune system. New studies indicate that it may be possible to direct the differentiation of human embryonic stem cells in cell culture to form insulin-producing cells that eventually could be used in transplantation therapy for diabetics. What a wonderful event this would be for the many people suffering from this debilitating disease.

To realize the promise of novel cell-based therapies for such pervasive and debilitating diseases, scientists must be able to easily and reproducibly manipulate stem cells so that they possess the necessary characteristics for successful differentiation, transplantation, and engraftment. The following is a list of steps in successful cell-based treatments that scientists will have to learn to precisely control to bring such treatments to the clinic.

To be useful for transplant purposes, stem cells must be reproducibly made to do the following:

* Proliferate extensively and generate sufficient quantities of tissue
* Not differentiate during this period of proliferation
* Differentiate into the desired cell type(s) upon selection
* Survive in the recipient after transplant
* Probably develop enzymes to hasten the action within the human body
* Integrate into the surrounding tissue after transplant
* Function appropriately for the duration of the recipient's life
* Present no serious side effects

Also, to avoid the problem of immune rejection, scientists are experimenting with different research strategies to generate tissues that will not be rejected. Adult stem cells that are pluripotent may prove to be valuable, since the body's rejection criteria will be reduced because they are from the same body.

To summarize, the promise of stem cell therapies is an exciting one, but significant technical hurdles remain that will only be overcome through years of intensive research. The last several years since 2007 have been very encouraging. It seems that that year began with some encouraging results, and they have increased rapidly since.

### Exciting News on Adult Stem Cells

There have been several dramatic discoveries recently about adult stem cells. An article appeared in *The Wall Street Journal* on November 15, 2007, written by Gautam Naik, discussing the results of a team of bio scientists under the leadership of Shoukhrat Mitalipov of the

Oregon National Primate Research Center. The team reported it had created monkey clones by using a variation of the process that yielded Dolly the sheep, the first cloned animal. This has to this point never occurred and is exciting, due to the similarity of the monkey genome to the human genome. This team wants to test whether fresh tissue derived from rhesus clones can treat diabetes or other diseases in a monkey, a process known as therapeutic cloning. Success in this process could strengthen future tests on humans. The idea is to create an embryonic clone of a patient, and then transplant altered versions of that embryo's cells back into the patient. I think it is important here to have the reader understand that the use of the word *clone* by this group may upset certain individuals who are against cloning. I think it is important to understand that this is a play on words. The other scientists working on embryonic stem cell research and adult stem cell research and those working on programming of cells are doing the same thing but calling it a different name. The group from Oregon actually worked with stem cells to generate their results and deliberately chose to use this wording. Ultimately, they want to create a complete monkey from embryonic stem cells, so as to be able to work with a subject that has been created from altered versions of the DNA of cells taken from this subject.

In their lab, they injected the genetic material from a skin cell of an adult monkey into a monkey egg whose own DNA had first been removed. This led to an early-stage embryo called a blastocyst, from which stem cells were then derived. Finally, they put the stem cells in a Petri dish and coaxed them into becoming long, thin nerve cells and beating heart tissue.

To show the difficulty in performing this experiment, the researchers used more than three hundred eggs from fourteen rhesus monkeys to derive their cell lines, which is fairly inefficient. I guess they learned as they proceeded, and future work would probably come at a better efficiency.

### Reports from Wisconsin and Japan

Two teams of scientists, one from Wisconsin and the other from Japan, have reprogrammed human skin cells so they are similar to embryonic stem cells, creating the promise of stem cell therapy without the need to destroy embryos. The article I got this information from is in the November 21, 2007, edition of the *San Jose Mercury News*.

The scientists started with normal human skin cells, hoping to induce them to become like human embryonic stem cells, which have the ability to turn into any type of tissue. Four genes suspected of causing pluripotency—the ability to turn into other types of cells—were implanted in retroviruses, which have the ability to insert genetic material into cell DNA. (See the section on AIDS, which is caused by the invasion of the DNA by a retrovirus that causes the DNA to have a new genetic code.) The skin cells were then exposed to the gene-carrying retroviruses. Within two weeks, the skin cells reverted to an embryonic state, becoming what is known as *induced pluripotent stem cells,* or *iPS cells.* The cells were then injected into mice, and the cells developed into a variety of tissue types, demonstrating that they had become pluripotent.

More research is needed; because retroviruses can cause cancer, researchers will likely need to find a way to insert the genes without the retroviruses.

The Yamanaka (Japan) team and the Wisconsin team that involved Thomson, the first to coax stem cells from human embryos in 1998, emphasized that more study is needed to determine if their reprogrammed cells are precisely like human embryonic stem cells. Scientists have long suspected that human embryonic stem cells contain a few key genes that give the cells pluripotency, the ability to become every tissue type. Through tests, the teams each picked four genes that seemed crucial to this capability. Then they added the genes to the skin cells along with a retrovirus, which can insert genetic material into a cell's DNA. After a couple of weeks, the cells became pluripotent. "Nobody has any idea the exact mechanism why these genes can actually turn skin cells back to human embryonic stem cell states" said Junying Yu, who led the Wisconsin team. But she suspects the genes turn on genetic material within the cells that helps convert the cells to an embryonic state.

Although both teams cautioned that more studies are needed to perfect the procedure, other experts proclaimed the accomplishments as a promising way to avoid the ethical debate surrounding human embryonic stem cells, which come from discarded embryos that are four to five days old.

This art of reprogramming seems to be moving fairly rapidly. I have now seen several articles where this method is being pursued—most of them with a great deal of early success. Even critics of stem cell research are endorsing this approach.

### Similar to My Computer Programs

I compare the similarity between this reprogramming method and the methods used in microprocessors and full computers. In computers, the inputs are decoded and recoded into what the computer wants to see (or is programmed to see). Data that the CPU manipulates are moved to the random access memory while the program is telling the CPU to do the next sequence. When this sequence is done (or many sequences), the information is then pulled from the random access memory (and may be placed in the memory again and fetched out with other data to give the full response needed), and the function is completed. The program for the computer is written in ROM (read-only memory), which normally cannot be erased; however, newer computer programs are now using read/write memories. The read is the active program, but certain data can result in the data telling the read/write to change to a write and take on a new program—in other words, create its own program based on data being received. If the data being received maintain a steady flow of similar information that the computer may not be programmed for, the data are then used to rewrite a change in the standard program to accommodate the most recent data.

Here's a rough example. Suppose a computer is programmed to handle information on temperatures being received that are between two temperature points. What if the data coming in continue to be strong enough to reprogram the computer to look at temperatures that are between two narrower temperature points, or if the opposite is true—to change the program to accept temperatures of a wider range? This is a form of self-programming.

Reprogramming cells requires a similar operation of "erasing" the present cell-stored program and rewriting the program to have the cell act in a different manner. In the case I just reviewed with you, they have essentially erased the DNA of the chromosomes and written in a new DNA code. The fact that a cell is shown to be able to accept this reprogramming and function with the new program is outstanding. The flaw so far is that they are using a retrovirus to do these functions. However, a retrovirus, as far as I can understand, is only a problem because it brings in "bad news," so to speak. I would expect that other means, either a retrovirus or a special RNA such as a coding RNA, will be developed to enter the cell and do the same functions as were done successfully by these two teams. I believe they used a retrovirus because they have already seen that a retrovirus (HIV) can enter a cell and change the code. In other words, this was the most straightforward way for them to try their methods. I believe what they have learned from these results establishes a great baseline for them, and this will place them in a position to go to the next step.

## My Thoughts

The one thing that remains a question in my mind is how long it would take for this method to take over a function of the body, such as a muscle function or the function of the pancreas to produce insulin of the correct amount. The reason for my question relates to what you have read in the section on HIV and how it enters the body. It does it by way of the retrovirus, but once done it takes many years for this HIV to replicate and cause the body to have AIDS—in some cases ten to twenty years. I would wonder how long it would take after reprogramming by the method being discussed for the human body to assimilate the new function; for example, take over the function of an arm muscle. I guess we will find out. I believe the key might be enzymes. As discussed, enzymes make things such as this to be accelerated—accelerated by a huge margin over waiting for nature to take its course. Some acceleration is in the billions over the normal time for a function to be done. Of course, designing an enzyme to do this function may not be simple. On the other hand, bio scientists have great experience on these types of requirements and may already have an enzyme in mind, based on their previous experiences. Hopefully, the enzyme selection will be straightforward. Remember, we learned that for every protein there is an enzyme. Maybe the body will produce the enzyme as the pluripotent reprogrammed cell is placed in the area for which it is designed.

### Pluripotent Stem Cells from Adult Skin Cells

The report in the newspapers on November 28, 2007, about the success in taking skin cells and reprogramming them to be pluripotent cells brought about a great deal of excitement. Television programs featured the woman doctor who worked on this procedure, and she was very excited. She said the tests done so far indicate the process works, and the cells were converted from differentiated skin cells to non-committed cells by "reprogramming the cells." This is the first time this has been accomplished. This has more implications than are obvious. The ability to reprogram cells from differentiated cells to non-committed cells that are pluripotent could open a very wide field of endeavor. I could assume that the ones for skin cells could definitely be used for providing new skin cells for a person in need of this type of cell, but, more importantly, if pluripotent as indicated, cells could be used for replacing cells in many places and eliminate the need for embryonic stem cells.

Maybe more importantly, remember when we discussed the normal cell and the genetic code and how the mRNA copies the DNA code in the nucleus and carries it out to the ribosome to have proteins generated? More recently, scientists have been able to change a codon on the code being carried by the mRNA to create the changed results they desired. Using the procedure just discussed to reprogram skin cells to be pluripotent appears to be an analogous situation. It even has more potential, since the pluripotent reprogrammed skin cells are undifferentiated. In theory, one should eventually be able to eliminate diseased sections of the body and introduce these pluripotent and reprogrammed stem cells into any given section of the body. The cells, since they were derived from the body, shouldn't have the rejection problems of other methods and should behave like a normal undiseased section of the body.

Another area of interest, which I may be way off base in mentioning, relates to AIDS and HIV, which are acquired through a retrovirus. The RNA of the retrovirus enters the nucleus of the cell and transcripts its code into the DNA of the cell. If the deprogramming method of skin DNA described in the newspapers could be directed toward the nucleus and DNA that has been changed by the HIV RNA; perhaps it could be deprogrammed to rid it of the contaminated DNA and convert it back to a healthy DNA. Wouldn't that be wonderful? It would prove out the method of deprogramming demonstrated by the bio scientists of the University of Wisconsin and those from Japan that reported on this method.

Of course we have to keep in mind that the standard programs on stem cells that have been in some level of force for a couple of years may prove to be the winner. These programs do not work on reprogramming standard body cells to become pluripotent. Instead, they work on the assumption that finding embryonic stem cells or developing them in vitro may be the most straightforward method of introducing the cells to the body without secondary problems. Remember, all these programs and various approaches are relatively new, and an advance in one direction may show what is needed to take it to the next step. The number of steps is not known yet. Whether one has reprogrammed cells that are pluripotent or embryonic cells that are omnipotent or adult cells that are found to be pluripotent, the scientists still have to determine the best way to introduce them to the human body. The first steps will be with mice and other animals. The recent favorable work with monkeys is a great step forward, since they have a genome that is similar to humans'.

## Scientists Are Meeting Their Objectives

With my limited knowledge, the "big deal" I see is that the programs are having the results that the people handling each of these diverse programs were expecting. This wasn't luck; it was the expected objective. This is significant, because there have been many approaches and all seem to provide the given researchers the results they were looking for. It's hard to ask for more than that from a new scientific program. Since there is so much experience with using stem cells from bone marrow to overcome some patients' leukemia, it would seem that one of these programs mentioned should be used in parallel with the present bone marrow transplant methods to give an informed result on a procedure with a history and determine if stem cells work the same or better. Rather than trying to find a person who can qualify as a donor, make a pluripotent stem cell that matches what is needed. It may show results faster and show where more work is needed. After all, bone marrow transplants are less than 50 percent successful at this time. Using omnipotent or pluripotent adult cells, or pluripotent reprogrammed cells, in place of the standard bone marrow from a matched donor may produce better results, and the people handling them would be more experienced in this transplant.

### Stem Cell Technique Cures Sickle-Cell Anemia in Mice

I read an article in the *San Jose Mercury News* on December 7, 2007, about a new technique developed by a research team from the Whitehead Institute for Biomedical Research in Cambridge, Massachusetts, and the University of Alabama at Birmingham, where scientists developed a new technique for curing sickle-cell anemia in mice by rewinding their skin cells to an embryonic state and manipulating them to create healthy genetically matched replacement tissue.

After the repaired cells were transfused into the animals, they soon began producing healthy blood cells free of the crippling deformities that deprive organs of oxygen.

The experiments, published online by the *Journal of Science*, confirmed the therapeutic potential of a new class of reprogrammed stem cells, which can be custom-made for patients without creating and destroying embryos. The strategy should work to treat hemophilia, thalassemia, and severe combined immunodeficiency disease—the "bubble boy" disease—according to researchers. Therapy might also apply to disorders linked to mutations in a single gene, such as muscular dystrophy and cystic fibrosis.

Scientists hope to use a similar approach to create cardiac cells to treat heart attack patients or nerve cells that could cure spinal cord injuries. Finding an abundant source of stem cells that could be used as a personalized biological repair kit is the goal of regenerative medicine.

The technique is a few years away from being used to treat humans, scientists said. Before it could be tried, several rounds of animal experiments would need to be done. But the study is certain to lure more researchers into studying the new class of induced pluripotent stem cells, or "iPS" cells. "There's going to be this 'tsunami,'" said Paul Simmons, director of the Center for Stem Cell Biology at the University of Texas Health Science Center in Houston. "One would have to predict that the pace of observations made using iPS cells is going to rise exponentially." These were my thoughts at the time; however, here we are eight years later and still trying to get to the results of a "tsunami." There has been progress, but there is much to learn. Perhaps there are too many alternatives and this spreads things thin. There are some results recently, and I will relate some.

This appears to be similar to the approach of making skin cells pluripotent, the work done by bio scientists at Wisconsin and in Japan, which I discussed earlier. This approach, if continued success follows, would leapfrog other approaches, since it works on deprogramming cells and making them "virgins" that haven't been differentiated. If a technique can remove the original DNA from a skin cell and produce pluripotent stem cells that can be used in various parts of the body, this provides super control, essentially depriving the original cell of its programming and allowing a reprogramming. It is like random access memories in computers that can be read and written and erased and rewritten. This means the bio scientists are learning how to communicate with the cells like the body communicates with the cells. Of course the "proof is in the pudding," as the saying goes. It has to be proved in humans. I believe that very shortly this can be tried in humans, perhaps those with no other chance of living. It will be similar to the story of Pasteur and his use of the cure for rabies on a child brought to him with no other chance of life except his serum. Let's hope this is tried on a human and is as successful as on a mouse. Remember, there is not much difference in the genome of a mouse compared to man.

### *Multiple Sclerosis Breakthrough.*

Here is a recent (early 2015) article from Stem Cell of America about the use of stem cells for multiple sclerosis treatment that shows a big advance over my basic write-up on stem cells. This is an article put out in the form of a recent report by Stem Cell of America (94)

### Multiple Sclerosis Treatment

### Treatment

The treatment performed at our clinics is a breakthrough medical procedure where Stem Cells (cellular building blocks) are usually administered intravenously and subcutaneously (under the skin) in Multiple Sclerosis patients. The whole procedure takes approximately one hour and has no known negative side effects.

No known negative side effects

Painless Procedure

Limited Space Available

Commonly, significant positive results are seen in three to six months.

Stem Cells will travel throughout the body, detecting damaged cells and tissue and attempts to restore them. The Fetal Stem Cells can also stimulate existing normal cells and tissues to operate at a higher level or function, boosting the body' own repair mechanisms to aid in the healing process. These highly adaptive cells then remain in the body, continually locating and repairing any damage they encounter.

### Safety

As with any medical treatment, safety should be of the highest priority. The Stem Cells used in our treatment undergo extensive screening for possible infection and impurities. Utilizing test more sophisticated than those regularly used in the United States for Stem Cell research and transplant. Our testing process ensures we use only the healthiest cells to enable the safest and most effective Fetal Stem Cell treatment possible. And, unlike other types of Stem Cells, there is no danger of the body's rejection of Fetal Stem Cells due to the fact they have no antigenicity (cellular fingerprint). This unique quality eliminates the need for drugs used to suppress the immune system, which can leave a patient exposed to serious infections.

### Results

With over 3000 patients treated, Stem Cell of America has achieved positive results with a wide variety of illnesses, conditions and injuries. Often, in cases where the diseases continued to worsen, our patients have reported substantial improvements following the Stem Cell treatment.

**Commonly, positive changes are seen between three to six months post treatment in Multiple Sclerosis patents.**

**To view follow-up letters from patients, please visit the** *patient experiences* page on our website.

Contact us to get more information on this breakthrough treatment.

### Disclaimer (by Stem Cell of America)

All statements, opinions, and advice on this page is provided for educational information only. It is not a substitute for proper medical diagnosis and care. Like all medical treatments and procedures, results may significantly vary and positive results may not always be achieved Please **contact us** so we may evaluate your specific case.

**My comments:** This is an outstanding treatment just like was suggested several years back on the use of stem cells. Results have been popping up in the newspapers, online, and in technical reports. Those readers interested in following the advances of stem cell results should visit websites on the computer or on their iPhone or other similar phones.

### Summary of Stem Cells

Keep in mind that stem cells were not discovered as such until the late 1990s and the adult stem cell around 2003. It has proved to be a long and detailed process with new discoveries on use that make them appear to be an answer, perhaps not as a direct use but in concert with other approaches—maybe problems being found in DNA research that will help to give a broader picture for their use. We have seen several significant successful steps taken since 2007 through to the present time on stem cell research. This has happened across a broad spectrum of research: on embryonic stem cells, on adult stem cells, and on programmed adult cells. Although there have been only recent advances on applying stem cells to humans, the use on different animals has proved very fruitful. As I previously commented, the encouraging thing is that every research experiment has resulted in the expected results. Probably the biggest advance was made in the reprogramming of cells to make them pluripotent. This ability, whether we use embryonic cells or adult cells or normal cells, gives us a major opportunity to deprogram cells and then reprogram them. If this continues to prove out, we may see many of the programs converge toward this approach. Even with available undifferentiated embryonic cells, researchers may not take the approach with these that has been used in the past. The reprogramming ability developed in the adult stem cell program should make it more straightforward to program embryonic cells, resulting from the synergy between programs.

It would appear that science has come up with a number of new weapons that will lead us toward applying the acquired knowledge on DNA and RNA, plus the use of stem cells, to combine into a broader program. It's one thing to be able to find the methods to obtain and use stem cells, but it will require the knowledge being gained on DNA and RNA to put this knowledge into effect. We may find that the knowledge we have learned during our battles with AIDS will prove valuable. Understanding the methods of rewriting DNA by the retrovirus has given some of the researchers the clues needed to develop stem cell programs that work similarly to the retrovirus. In one case, programming of bacteria used a retrovirus to obtain the results. It would seem the key thing to be pursued in the near future is to figure out how to program RNA to act like a retrovirus and enter the cell nucleus and become part of the genome of the body, without the concern that the retrovirus might bring HIV with it. Since we have discovered in other battles with cancer that the use of a virus allows us to focus the chemical treatments on the exact location of the cancer, we may find that we can use a virus in the same manner to carry the RNA into the nucleus. Likewise, there may be some synergy with the attack on cancer using some of the techniques developed in the stem cell programs. The programs on genetics, stem cell research, AIDS, DNA, and RNA seem to be converging with each bit of knowledge we gain. I am eighty-three years of age and hope that I get to see the fruitful completion of these programs, with some part of a human body being generated through some of the technologies mentioned and replaced successfully in a human being. It's time to get off the mouse and onto humans. It's in the cards and just a matter of when.

# The Wonders of Extending Life

I have taken you from early life several hundred years ago, from the time when the Great Famine occurred, followed by the Black Death and onward, through the various phases of life and its various transformation battles and battles with various medical problems and solutions. Man has been aided by the sun and its constant energy to provide the elements and energy needed by both to make this a successful journey. The bio scientists and doctors fought long and tenuous battles, with some methods provided by nature to defend ourselves other than just the use of our brains. Man has learned how to fight the various battles successfully and to take some control over nature into his own hands. This story has shown that, for man to survive, he had (and has) to depend on others to combine their energies and work together to provide the basics needed for life to continue successfully. However, as we have seen, man has been his worst enemy as well, and this resulted in many wars that brought significant loss of human life. The good news—man took advantage of what he learned during these wars. The fight against many ailments, including infection and those carried by insects or animals, were fought and won during and after the wars. Meanwhile, the many patients to work on provided considerable experience and the opportunity to work on many new technologies discovered during the wars and immediately after. It's a shame, but wars provide many opportunities in a short period of time, and the wonderful opportunity for many to be involved in the same objects—peace and good health.

There have been huge catastrophes over the years, as spelled out in my coverage of the five worst ones, along with the many wars, and man has survived—usually profiting from some new advances in technology developed during the wars. Man's ingenuity seemed to increase as he prepared for the various wars, using his brains to fight a new foe under different conditions. Maybe the major improvements found during wars result from many people focusing their energies together to solve a common problem for all—fighting a war and gaining peace. It's the one time when the people of whole countries are focused and working together to resolve a problem with less politics involved.

It is in the role of advocate, man to man, that man has made the greatest progress. During the years that have passed, man has learned how to educate himself and use this education as his biggest weapon. He learned how to spread this education during wars, during the movements of different religions, and eventually through the written and printed word through the development of the alphabet and the invention of the printing press. Thus began the use of mass communication through books. As man ventured to other parts of the earth, he carried this education with him as he went on his way. Today man has additional powerful tools to help fight the battle, including computers and mass communication through the use of iPads and iPhones (or their equivalents supplied by others). Science has rapidly advanced and provided medical tools that are wonders that were not here twenty or thirty years ago. Precision tools have been generated that make operations possible with less damage occurring as a result of the operation. A person working on a problem and finding a solution can pick up his iPhone and talk to the right people anywhere in the world in less than two minutes, telling them what he has found and how he found it. He may be giving the clue to those people on how that could help them to solve a completely different problem. The wonders of mass communication have speeded up the advances of medical achievements and vice versa.

Early on, many of man's battles were against the silent foes of disease and pestilence. Not having any background or education on the cause of diseases resulted in high percentages of human life being expended. It is one of the wonders of life that man has been able to survive the terrible plagues and huge wars, including two world wars that struck without a reasonable cause. Man was perhaps fortunate in many of those plagues, since he had no knowledge on how to overcome them; yet they went away for reasons unknown in many cases. At times plagues would return, and man first learned to quarantine the sick from the healthy as the first major advance against the silent killers. The wonders developed by the technical world helped to carry life forward even though mass quarantine still remains a huge start toward overcoming the issue. Today's situation with Ebola in western North Africa is a prime example where quarantine is still being used today. Advanced experiences during these times allowed man to become educated on how to fight many of these silent enemies, later to be followed by technical advances to finish the job. There have been many learning curves for human beings as we made this journey through time to the present day.

The nineteenth century proved to be a very powerful century in the battles against bacteria. The advent of the microscope, allowing the genius of man to see the enemy and see what affected these small enemies, was a monstrous achievement, led by a Dutch janitor. We began to see our medical heroes appear. People like Pasteur, Koch, Lister, and many others shared in establishing what caused the various diseases and, in most cases, how to overcome the diseases. In some cases enemies were observed under the microscope, but there were no miracle drugs to help to overcome them. Man found that certain diseases were caused by certain mosquitoes and certain flies, and this allowed for the battle to be fought and generally won by man. Man's makeup allowed for survival in many cases. Implementing the methods of improved hygiene on an everyday basis and in the operating room began to prevent certain diseases and keep them from spreading. Documentation became a valuable asset as we learned more and more about the microbes that could cause us harm and how to overcome them, as they could be recorded for movement onto the next step of survival of the human race.

As the nineteenth century came to a close, there were many technical advances besides medical ones. Man's ingenuity began to be asserted. The steam engine provided a power source for transportation and equipment. Rail lines were installed across the United States, allowing locomotives to ship supplies across the country, as well as providing a means of travel for people. Steam-driven boats carried the many supplies needed for such things as the production of steel. These steam-driven beauties floated across the Great Lakes and down the many rivers of America to their final destinations to deliver their goods. Steam was king, and many advances followed—sort of waiting for the next big advancement in the means of transportation.

Then came a new king—oil. The first oil wells were drilled for commercial use by Drake in Titusville, Pennsylvania, in the later parts of the nineteenth century. Man used this energy to create new power tools and equipment. This expanded the capabilities for many things, including the plowing of fields for more food crops and to prevent another Great Famine. Then the first automobiles were built in small numbers at the end of the century. Tesla and George Westinghouse gave the United States the AC power needed to power machinery and provide man with a source of energy. Electric power initially came from places like Niagara Falls, with its natural drop to the river below, which was converted into a source of electrical power. Long transmission lines began to be laid to provide access to electric power to remote locations across the United States and many other countries of the world. The telegraph gave us a means of long-distance communication. Edison invented mass production and use of the lightbulb, one of the wonders of life that helped to extend man's day. Now man could see during the dark of evening and gain additional time to solve problems or produce needed materials. It's difficult to imagine how many things were done years ago when there were no electric lights for the doctors and advancers of technology to see. Edison's light gave them visibility, and his phonograph gave many the chances to listen to sounds they had never heard before.

At the turn of the twentieth century, many of man's contributions were involved in the Industrial Revolution. The Wright brothers flew the first airplane in 1903 and worked out the bugs on advanced designs that were used by the military in the years that followed. The evolution of the airplane was swift; many were produced in the years to follow. Henry Ford introduced the automobile production lines that would allow the average person to own an automobile. This provided many new outlets for man in his search for entertainment, as well as another transportation option for factory materials and the ability of people to drive to work many miles away from their homes. These were the obvious results, but the unseen results of the medical industry and its technical counterparts were not obvious until proved later: and they were proved.

Albert Einstein produced four amazing papers in 1904 that gave man a better view of the world and the universe. Several scientists were involved in the development of the basic knowledge of how atoms work, with Niels Bohr being one of the main contributors. There was World War I, which again pitted man against himself. The wonders of life became the weapons of war and meant death to many—but not all by bullets. Many were claimed by infectious diseases caused by *Staphylococcus* and *Streptococcus* bacteria. We have discussed the development of the sulfa drugs that allowed man to battle these two bacteria, to almost a complete victory. When the sulfa drugs began to lose their potency, English scientists and American pharmaceutical companies did significant work to provide penicillin to fight these diseases and others. These truly were the wonders of life.

And then in midcentury came another traumatic war—World War II, which saw almost the whole world involved in some way in this war. During the war many technical achievements arrived, including the first jet airplanes near the end of the war. Synthetic materials were invented and developed throughout many industries, providing man sources of new materials. These would yield added warmth in the cold weather, improved tires for automobiles and airplanes, lighter materials for certain applications, easier materials to mold into new forms, material that wouldn't rust, and new fabrics for clothes to wear. The synthetics would also provide man with other means of developing medicines for fighting germs in one way or another. DDT was used to nearly rid the world of malaria until man learned of its side effects.

Near the end of the war the atomic bomb was developed, which magnified the early-century genius of Einstein into a horrendous form of energy to both help and hurt mankind. We learned how to use atomic power for energy to supply electricity and to develop some forms of it to provide radioactive markers for mapping the happenings going on inside our bodies. Commercial jet planes that had twice the speed of the propeller-driven planes and flew at over twice the altitude took over worldwide transportation and provided means of supplying materials and food to many parts of the world. All of these improvements in transportation helped the medical community supply needs to the ailing in one way or another. To the people of the world, the planet started looking like a smaller place. The world began acting as one community, with each country realizing its capabilities and spreading them the world over. Now each country was a resource, and the other countries recognized this capability to contribute, either through uniqueness or the ability to use its resources in a better fashion. The world got smarter relative to the rules of supply and demand. We now had a world where one country could supply from its capabilities through exports and receive other country's capabilities through imports to help balance the needs of the world.

The genius of man then brought television to the people of the world, first in black and white, and then in color. Now we could watch the people in "real time" in all parts of the world or watch a ball game instead of having to buy a ticket to a game. About this time Jonas Salk developed the polio vaccine, which essentially eliminated poliomyelitis (polio) disease from the world and made swimming in public pools by children the world over possible again. The flu vaccine was developed, which has to be renewed each year to provide immunity for the annual seasonal flu mutations; but the ingenuity of man discovered how to handle this mutation, and it works—people are treated again to another wonder of life. During the century other vaccines for multiple diseases were developed and put into mass production to provide for the world over.

Late in the forties the transistor was invented by the people of Bell Labs. This provided a new means of handling signals and reducing the power needed by radios and televisions and many other appliances. They were minute in size and more rugged and used less power. As a result, most electronic equipment became smaller and more portable and lasted longer. Now man could walk around with equipment and watch or listen to what was going on in the world on a "real time" basis. From this beginning came the integrated circuits and the next step up in electronics. Electronic equipment became a partner in the war against pestilence and offered unique solutions to medical procedures. (I was awarded the Distinguished Alumni Award from the University of Pittsburgh in 2012 for having invented the first single-chip silicon analog integrated circuit in 1959.) The technological world was advancing as rapidly as the world's needs to fight other elements that stood in the way of man's progress. It seemed as though it was a race, since as one element was overcome it seemed as though another popped up. It seemed as if as man got older he moved into another area of medical problems or expansion of old problems due to the large increases in population around the world.

After considerable study and work by scientists the world over, next would come answers to the riddles of man and his genetics. These wonders had been sought since man could talk and think. This latest search started in the nineteenth century and continued in the twentieth century right up to the present time. Scientists first discovered deoxyribonucleic acid (DNA) and ribonucleic acid (RNA) in the chromosomes early in the nineteenth century, but they did not consider these to be part of the heritage and secrets of life. This soon would be resolved.

It was determined that all forms of life, including plants, animals, and man, are made up of cells. After World War II, the drive to find how man inherits his various characteristics was continued in earnest. It was a drive to determine our genetic makeup, given the exciting name "the genetic code." The world of science began to search for the genetic code. Chromosomes—twenty-three pairs of them— were discovered in every cell of the human body, and scientists soon knew that they provided the source of genetics and the genetic code, but science couldn't determine how this was achieved. Researchers believed the key was in the DNA of the chromosomes within the nucleus of human cells, but needed to find how this hidden code inside this nucleus worked. In 1952, the main part of the answer came.

An American, James D. Watson, and two Englishmen, Maurice Wilkins and Francis Crick, along with Rosalind Franklin, who provided the amazing X-ray images of DNA, determined that DNA was a double helix, which is shaped like a spiral staircase, with base pairs between the rungs of the staircase, like stair steps. The strings of base pairs, like the rungs of a ladder between the double helix backbones determine the genetic code of the person. Watson and Crick also determined how DNA works, providing—via RNA—triplets of information that leave the nucleus via messenger RNA. This sequence provides information that activates various amino acids and builds the proteins that are required by the human body from these acids. These codes and their resultant actions provide twenty of the twenty-two Amino acids needed by man. The other two must be supplied by consuming the proper food.

It is worth mentioning that computers became a huge technical entity around the mid-twentieth century and played an important part in almost every form of activity that man was involved in. Computers, along with the appropriate programs, became the main problem-solving instruments. The evolution of the computer—from the use of vacuum tubes to transistors and eventually to integrated circuits, along with increased speed and size reduction—was probably the biggest technical achievement in the second half of the twentieth century. This involved the transition from the use of transistors to the use of integrated circuits in 1959; various types of transistors completed circuit functions, rather than the simple functions of transistors. Without the computers to do fast calculations and provide answers rapidly, many of the designs of man and of nature would have been hard to come by. The computer was to solving many problems like an enzyme was to proteins; it speeded up the answers. It also served to allow man to operate in remote places, taking man's place in environments not people-friendly, such as outer space and deep underground (when looking for oil) or deep in the oceans (when looking for anything that would advance man). When reviewing the achievements of man during the last half of the twentieth century, I find it hard to find one that didn't use the computer in some way to give refined results at super speeds. Man was on a roll with the aid of computers and microprocessors, and this roll was joined by the bio scientists and others of the medical community.

Man conquered "near" outer space as space vehicles were designed, and man made his first adventures around the earth in these unique spacecraft in the late 1950s. Then man made the trip to outer space, beginning space flights in the late 1950s. The United States sent man to the moon and back in 1968. It was exciting to see earth from a distance, and it looked like we had thought it would. Here was this wondrous planet that I have written about. It appeared as a handsome figure when viewed from the moon. Here man stood on the moon, which had been created early in the life of earth when a collision of some space debris hit earth—and now it serves to provide us a view from either object, the earth or the moon. It also provides us the valuable light each night so things can be accomplished as they have been since the time of man.

It's worth mentioning that man had found how to capture some of the energy from the sun with an invention called the solar cell. It was this invention that now provided energy to the space vehicles, with their clear view of the sun. Man found that the vacuum of space was ideal to fan out the solar cell array in a sail-like extension from the space vehicle to soak up the sun, without being concerned about wind blowing against the energy cells. The vacuum of outer space provides man with no source of oxygen for his needs, and so these are supplied by the manufacture of oxygen using the power of the solar cell to operate unique equipment inside the vehicle to provide the needed oxygen. All the advances in reducing the size and increasing the capabilities of electronics were utilized throughout the space vehicle. These same capabilities developed for these trips to outer space provided additional capabilities for medical advancements and improving the health of the people of the world.

In the early 1980s came good and bad news for mankind. The good news was in the form of small computers using microprocessors that evolved into the personal computer (PC) marketplace. The size of computers decreased while their computer power increased; and this evolution resulted in a large part of the world's population having personal computers to use as they so choose. The bad news was the arrival of the HIV virus and the resultant AIDS, which was a sentence to death. It was later determined that the virus was brought into the country in 1969 from the island of Haiti, although its origin was determined to be Africa. I have covered this extensively in prior sections of this book. Men and women the world over work on solutions for those that have the HIV virus to prevent the development of AIDS and the death that follows. Where at one time HIV would turn into full-blown AIDS in several years, the medical profession has increased the life span of those with HIV and delayed AIDS for twenty years and for a lifetime for many. The world of HIV and AIDS gave the scientific world a better understanding of how the RNA and DNA work in the human body. Much has been accomplished to prevent HIV and to extend the life of those involved. Meanwhile, it gives the present workers in stem cell technology considerable advanced information on how things work inside the cells of the body and how to approach many of their experiments. Knowledge begets knowledge.

Over the 1980s, 1990s, and on into the new century, the personal computer shrank in size per function performed and gained higher speeds and new programs for solving problems, as well as providing huge storage capacity. These small computers, about one-hundredth the size of the large computers of the 1950s, have more memory than the huge computers of the 1970 variety. Many new companies were started around the world using the PC format with Microsoft's software. Intel was the biggest supplier of the microchips for the microprocessor; Microsoft supplied the software. Apple Computer was the biggest competitor with the PC, with its unique software and hardware. The biggest PC supplier was Dell Computer in Texas, but Hewlett-Packard passed them in 2006. It turns out that all of these companies still produce the computer, and some the fast printers that are available. The knowledge gained on these soon brought on advancements in equipment that acted like computers but could be carried in a smaller format, like the iPads and iPhones and equipment like this supplied by many the world over.

The peripheral gear for the computer, including the printer, the fax machine (which allowed one to send printed material electronically to anywhere in the world), and the copier allowed the home computer person to do most of the functions required by many industries and transfer the information via the computer or the fax. The home now essentially had more computing power and peripheral capability than the industrial computers of the 1970s and early 1980s. We did not have to go to a library to read a book; it was on the electronics of this age. We did not have to write a letter and send it through the mail, because we could do it on the Internet via our computers, or our cell phones, or our iPads; life was fun.

At the end of the 1980s or in the early 1990s, a means of using the home computer to communicate around the world was invented: the Internet and the World Wide Web. This brought communication to another level, which exceeded the telephone in many cases. One of the biggest advantages of this means of communication was during massive emergency situations such as earthquakes and tsunamis. One could send an e-mail to the emergency area, and they didn't have to respond to it like they do with a telephone. The message would be downloaded on the receiving end, and the e-mail could be addressed at the convenience of those in the disaster area or on a priority basis. Administrators of hospitals could review the list of download messages and select which ones were more important. This capability allowed them to not have to answer all phone calls, some of which were not critical. It also provided the sender the knowledge that he or she had sent the message and that sooner or later it would be answered. This was much better than hearing a busy signal on a telephone and having to hang up and keep trying later. I have given one example, but there are millions of other examples.

These small computers and their capabilities allowed the space vehicles to be functional and to monitor their space capability at all times. Communication from these vehicles was carried out by the onboard computers, and the space vehicle was controlled in many cases by earth-stationed computers that provided information to the onboard computers. Man really had conquered how to function away from the mother planet. Now came such things as the drones—a technical form of an airplane but without a pilot—that could do good or do some bad. Here was the equivalent of small airplanes that could see via the computer and other electronics and resolve what they saw via a remote computer thousands of miles away.

The books I have written, including this one, use all of these capabilities, which allow me to look up data in minutes that would require days or weeks if I had to go to libraries and search out the information. The Internet and World Wide Web gave me access to information that no encyclopedia could provide and most libraries do not have at their disposal. With this advance, the world became another level smaller, because one could communicate with almost any place in the world just by sitting down at home on the PC and using the Internet, the fax machine, or the cell phone, and do it inexpensively—many at no cost at all.

Cell phones, which allowed a person to talk to anyone around the world, arrived in the 1980s. These cell phones began to methodically shrink in size and expand in capability. In many cases they allowed the capability of seeing other people, perhaps thousands of miles away, on an LCD display while talking to them. Perhaps the biggest impact they had was in countries like China, India, Malaysia, and other countries in the Far East without the telephone lines and power lines that existed in the Western world. Their job—to keep up with the progress in the West—was a monstrous one when one considers the work they had to do to provide this asset. This would have required many thousands of miles of digging to install telephone poles and transmission lines. Then came wireless cell phones, and these countries could put off the monstrous task of supplying the infrastructure for basic communication needs, including such things as telephone poles that would have had to cross the countries. Now all they had to do was build cell phone centers at strategic locations, and before you knew it they were in business and communicating with the rest of the world. Several billion people were turned on to advanced communication. People the world over became walking pieces of communication equipment.

Soon, these cell phones became outdated and were replaced with more sophisticated electronics. They are being supplanted by the iPhone or the equivalent. This also proved to be a winner, since the new phones were smaller and lighter, and could provide programs that are on computers. People not only carried telephones but had direct communication with the Internet and its vast means of communication and information, supplying answers to questions that one had to previously look through an encyclopedia to find. These small phones and their capabilities could be used for navigation, watching the stock market, sending text messages to anywhere in the world at no cost, taking pictures, used as a phone, used to replace one's home computer, and invention goes on at this time in late July of 2015

Meanwhile in the 1990s, new approaches to cameras for the consumer became a big item. These cameras used solid-state CCD (charge coupled device) memories for storing the picture instead of film; later flash memories would invade this field. Digital cameras became smaller, with greater capability, and could be carried in pockets or purses; and, of course, on one's iPhone.

Stick (or thumb) memories became a big item in the first years of the twenty-first century. Small products called stick memories were packaged in a plastic or metal package that was about a quarter-inch thick, half an inch wide, and one to four inches long, and they held memories that were bigger than the entire memories of the big computers of the 1990s. They became the chief means for transferring information from one computer to another and could be carried from one place to another or used to store electronic records of such things as pictures, books, and anything that could be provided by the PC. They relieved the computer memories so they could continue to navigate the real-time action, and it was stored forever. All of these technologies were the benefactors of the digital process, which had begun to take over the functions of analog devices in the 1960s. I was one of the first inventors of the silicon integrated circuit, later called the chip, and did much work in the analog and digital worlds of integrated circuits. As the twentieth century came to a close, television sets began to be introduced in a digital mode. It proved easier to design circuits for a specific function and easier, eventually, to receive the information. The way was now open to design systems that were completely digital, were faster, used less power, and were less expensive to use.

Early in the 2000s, companies like Apple began delivering—in one small, compact size, comparable to a pack of cigarettes—a combination cell phone, camera, extensions to one's computer, access to music, access to movies, access to any video, access to the stock market, and, probably more importantly, allowed the user to communicate with the Internet. There are many other functions that are too extensive for me to list here. All these forms of communication—the cell phone, the computer, the Internet, the fax machine, the printer, the solid-state camera, the television, the advanced transmission lines, and many other electronic wonders— allowed the world to become quite close. It was nothing to transmit business information or entertainment from one's home to others thousands of miles away via these new, fast, sharper, simpler, and broader means of information, as if they were in the next room.

This is just the beginning. I will give you a personal experience that occurred in our family. My niece's youngest son (about thirteen at the time) awakened with a terrible headache in 2005. He was flown to a major hospital in Pittsburgh, Pennsylvania, where they found that an artery had broken in his brain. They had no way of handling this, but they had information that Johns Hopkins in Baltimore had developed new glue that would allow repair of this type of break. They contacted Johns Hopkins, and they began to take steps immediately to solve the problem. They flew the glue to Pittsburgh, and the doctors there were directed by television on how to apply the glue. This performance began while the doctors from Johns Hopkins watched via the television and advised the doctors in Pittsburgh. The operation was a success, but the following day the bleeding reappeared and the doctors from Pittsburgh performed the operation a second time. My grandnephew didn't go to school for about a year and then began to take classes and almost caught up before he graduated. During these years he had problems with one leg and walking and problems with the use of his left arm. Meanwhile, Botox, a terrible poison capable of poisoning the world with a teaspoon if used that way, was developed to remove problems that people had with eyes and other physical ailments. In 2010 my grandnephew was given a special shot of this Botox type of medicine in his leg and arms. By 2012 he had a slight limp and improved use of his arm. Keep in mind how toxic this Botox was only several years ago, yet the bio scientists were able to find how to process it and use it to their advantage. Here is a family experience that used the technologies developed to help his major brain problem to the present time. Many medical and technical advances have saved this person's life, and I am sure this type of progress is going on all over the world.

## *Why the Technical Entities?*

Why did I shift my discussion to these technical entities? I want the reader to realize there were advances in other things besides medicine and gaining knowledge about man's genetic makeup. Also, technical innovations became the backbone of the medical industry in finding solutions to diseases. I want the reader to have a feel for the vast knowledge that man has created to provide a more international means of communicating to the people around the world and to focus vast resources to the culmination of finding the genetic code and the stem cell. One could now swallow a camera that was very small; as it made its way through the body, it gave the viewer a complete view on a screen of the trail of this small electronic wizard, from the throat to the ejection at the end of the trip. Medical people could now see what went on in the body, from the mouth all the way through the digestive system and to completion. They could definitely find the problem and more definitely find the solution to the medical problem that related to the path of this electronic wizard. There were now magnetic resonant imaging devices (MRIs) that scanned the body using this system, bit by bit. From the scan, computers and other electronics converted these data into a three-dimensional picture of whatever part of the body the doctors chose to review. One could see brain images as no other piece of equipment could show them—in three dimensions. There were now ultrasonic scans that would allow the doctors to view the functions inside the body just by moving this small (about the size of a man's fist) instrument across the part of the body they wanted to scan. This instrument is noninvasive, inexpensive for the patient, and easy for the doctor's assistants to run as they view on a monitoring TV screen in real time whatever they want to scan; you find the results within several minutes. They can review the functioning of a person's blood flow through the carotid arteries in the neck and see if there are any impediments to the flow. Ultrasound makes it easy to check for kidney stones, carotid artery blockage issues, aortic aneurisms, and other organ functions of the body. Women have their breasts checked for breast cancer through the use of mammograms that provide a picture of the internal parts of the breast. This allows for early detection and early medical involvement in eliminating these tumors. These are all instruments of life to prevent death.

One of the most outstanding features of the progress made in surgical methods relates to the fact that many operations can now be performed without making major incisions in the body. Small, unique, and precise equipment allows operations to be performed through very small incisions that allow specialized equipment to enter the area to perform surgery. New blood tests were developed that could check a man's PSA, which is an indication if prostate cancer is a problem. New equipment could perform a colonoscopy via the rectum to determine if he or she has polyps, which are growths that could be cancerous or the start of cancer. Polyps can then be removed with the same piece of equipment. Various new portable equipment is available that is inexpensive and provides a means for a person to monitor his or her blood pressure. Many different blood pressure medicines were developed by the pharmaceutical companies to treat individuals for hypertension. Individuals could monitor their own blood pressure quite easily on an hour-by-hour basis, if necessary, to determine whether the new medicine was performing its required function. Likewise for people suffering from high blood sugar—equipment is available for puncturing the skin on one's finger and checking the blood for the sugar level while one is sitting at home.

Radiation and chemotherapy were now the methods of choice for attacking cancer. The chemotherapy that is now being developed is designed to work on a given organ of the body. This customized and focused approach to attack a given type of cancer is being developed by small and large pharmaceutical companies the world over. Year by year, they develop new synthetic compounds to ward off the various cancers, sometimes focused by the use of a virus that can penetrate the given cells in the targeted organ and carry these chemicals into the desired area.

I have written about the successful method of taking a polio virus, and through electronic control, placing it exactly on a cancerous tumor, and having the combination of this virus penetrating the tumor surface and one's immune system eventually eliminate the cancerous tumor.

I've discussed the use of our experience with DNA, RNA, stem cells, and AIDS, and which genes control which portion or portions of the body. We are beginning to see how the human body itself has been evolving through evolutionary methods to better protect the body. We used to believe evolution took thousands of years, but we are beginning to see that it happens in hundreds of years, and in some cases real time. We have seen how enzymes in our body accelerate chemical reactions that take seconds, but would take thousands of years if it weren't for these enzymes. Now we are working on chemicals that enhance actions within the body to give us medical information that would take many years using past methods. We will find many new methods as we keep gaining knowledge on the wonders of life. (I hope you noticed that I changed the singular word. I think of it as a wonder, but it's probably wonders.)

So, now you see why I included some information about electronics. I wanted to be sure that you were aware of man's battles against the silent killers that we call microbes and how they are being assisted by the smallest of electronics, which we call microcircuits or chips. Man has come a long way since I started writing about his appearance on earth. To think that life was started by some DNA or RNA that became DNA about a half million years ago and evolved into man, makes life more a wonder. Prehistoric man came without any built-in weapons to fight for his survival besides a keen mind, his strength, and the ability to use other things that were available. He has used this keen mind to make him the "head of the food chain," so to speak. Just twenty-three hundred years ago, the world was populated by three hundred million humans. The earth's population was 1.2 billion people 150 years ago, and now it is 7.25 billion people—all of which speaks for man's ability to survive. Of course, earth had much to do with it. It evolved into a better place to live through its acquisition of the various needs for man's survival. And then there's the sun, which made it possible for these transformations to take place. The sun adopted this planet as its own and helped to sculpt it into the place we now know. It was fun writing about the success of man (and woman) through the many cycles of nature's attacks on us humans. Mother Nature is the only thing that has come close to closing the book on man. However, as the years proceeded and man's learning curve brought new knowledge to the forefront, man has learned some ways to overcome the challenges of Mother Nature. It seems that the biggest threat to man is man himself.

## Conclusion

I named this book *Life and Death* because I felt it was a wonder that man has survived and can look back and see the obstacles he has overcome and the knowledge he has gained—not only about the world, but also about himself and how his internal system works. It's a wonder how the puzzle pieces were put together and developed by man as time proceeded. Initially I was writing about the tough times man lived through and how he survived them; then all of a sudden there was a shift in my writing to man's advancements and his advantages. It was like man went from a defensive battle to an offensive one. This major change probably occurred during the middle of the 1800s, when the microscope allowed man to see the little things we couldn't see without it. Here was a shift in the battle—if we could see it, we could defeat it. This offensive battle continued with the development of tools that bio scientists and medical doctors could use to improve their success rates and improve detailed operations. This offensive approach was clearly evident as man refined the elements that came together to provide him a glance at DNA and the details that made it work. This became the human genome, spread like a map before us, which we could now start analyzing, sticking a pin (not really, but it acted like this) in the various gene sites to see which ones affected which parts of our human system. We now had a road map, where a generation ago we were blindfolded. It took years to develop the first genome of man. Today, many genomes can be done in a single day. Being able to supply a genome within a day is like providing a picture of a person's life within the time needed to keep his life ... alive. This is a recent miracle. At one time it took a couple of years to do a person's genome. Now, with today's equipment we could not only see it in a day but review it over a few days and determine where a problem occurs, and in some cases find a solution to the problem. Science keeps moving forward and faster these days. In addition, the knowledge is passed around the world almost immediately. Faster communication has been responsible for many of today's advances in medicine and physical issues.

It's interesting when you consider that we have just arrived on this road map of the human genome. We have inched up on it. Like all road maps, the more you use them the more real they become. I can imagine the impact of the human genome on the world of scientists and doctors of all types. I believe with the aid of the genome and the use of computers the world over that we will find a rapid way to map the specific genomes of the individuals with certain diseases and see what is common in their genomes. From this, medical science will discover how to affect a given gene to resolve a given issue. This will transform from a research methodology on individuals to resolution of man's everyday general ills. The "back and forth" method of reviewing genomes and relating and comparing information about others with certain comparable unique capabilities in rapid time allows doctors to make different decisions today than they would have made two years ago.

We will work that genetic code for more information that will lead us to things one could not predict as short a time ago as 2013, and may be able to predict at this time. There are plenty of predictions, and many of them will be proved true. I am talking about what we don't know and can't predict at this time. With every finding come many surprises. The good news is that man has learned to document his findings so the surprises have a road map under way. In addition, the computer is both the method of documentation and the key to solving problems. One of my engineers said to me about thirty years ago, "Computers can only do what you program them to do. They are basically dumb." To which I answered, "You are right to a certain degree, but as you use the computer and it brings back answers, it also shows you what is not the answer. This allows one to think about the right answer and apply different information into the computer.

When this is applied to the computer, a new solution arrives, and it does this so rapidly and exactly that it allows one to have information he didn't have only minutes ago. So, as dumb as it is, it makes the user smarter. Therefore, the result is one of gained intelligence that one could not have without the computer in a given time frame."

I believe the human genome will eventually be placed on a computer with a proper program that will allow real-time active intervention. You will be able to change one gene slightly, and the computer will feed back information about how that affects other genes. This will allow interactive play between the scientists and the simulated genome in the computer. As this type of action and reaction occurs, it will teach the scientist what affects what within this genome. The initial attempts at this will not work as smoothly as one would like, but it gives the user and programmer some answers that lead to improved models, and it does it rapidly. This will continue to evolve into a magnificent tool for the solution of many medical problems. One must realize when he is using a computer that it contains the inputs from many people, including many engineers, many programmers, many computer scientists, many mathematicians, many scientists, and many bio scientists, plus your own input as you use it. So you are not working with a dumb machine; you are working with the best of the best. The wonder of the computer and present-day rapid communication brings information around the world; so we get to see the best of the best.

I have shown the similarities between the HIV virus and the DNA/RNA workings, and I believe there will be a continuing of dramatic results on curing HIV and AIDS within a few years. Perhaps it will also provide the answers for Ebola, since AIDS is only one of many retroviruses that attack the human system. A solution to any one of the retroviruses will result in feedback to solve other ones. The ability to program skin cells to be omnipotent or pluripotent leads me to believe that a similar action will occur with HIV and AIDS. Since the HIV virus inserts itself into the DNA (much like the RNA injects itself inside the nucleus to be programmed by the DNA) and causes the rewriting of the person's DNA—such that each cell in the body eventually has this new DNA with this devilish new program—I believe that in the not too distant future we will find a way to reprogram the infected DNA and remove the retrovirus signature. We have to find a way to write the HIV virus's program to make it null and void. If this can be caught early in the cycle of the infection by the HIV virus, we should be able to erase it. There is no doubt that once a person has AIDS, the problem is much tougher. That would involve erasing every cell in the human body. Since it takes years for HIV to progress to AIDS, it may take that long to undo it. However, I think not. There must be one cell in the human body that has the "chief DNA" in it, and when we find it we will make one change and the whole body will begin to change its DNA. There have been recent accomplishments on the curing of HIV. Bio scientists have combined two or more medications that had some effects on HIV when used alone, and they recently combined several and have had positive effects. So we may be almost there?

I believe this review of history, including today's advances, does a good job of showing the reader how man's technology did a great job of finding out how to deal with the silent and unseen bearers of disease and death and on how rapidly today's technology is making some of them disappear or to be tolerable. This battle with bacteria and viruses has been a long one, but man has persevered. The battle went from one of being a passive finder of the silent and unseen to one of an active one, where man has been able to provide an even better picture and is now preempting some before the fact. The better understanding of the genome and where the genes do their jobs will bring even more positive action in the near future. Stem cells will allow us to repair parts of our body that malfunction, and life should be extended well beyond the present length. We can now see the unseen, and it is no longer silent—and neither is man as he continually invokes his repairs.

I hope this review of the tough times that man has endured will make it easier for the reader to understand what it takes to continue this journey and keep improving it. When you consider work on the genome occurred over about sixty years, it didn't take long once we got a glimpse of how the genetic code works. It took us a couple thousand years to get to that point. I am sure there is tons more to learn, but it continually provides a daily exciting adventure.

After completing this book, I thought maybe I should have called it *The Wonders of Life*, rather than *Life and Death*, since it is obvious that a plural is involved when considering life. Life is wondrous, even when it's tough. The good news is that it is only tough when you're living through it, but it's a piece of cake when you look back. That's what I am doing now. Are you?

John Durbin Husher

# About The Author

John Durbin Husher was born as a twin in 1932 with his twin brother Lee Kenneth Husher. They were born in Monessen Pennsylvania.

Graduated from Monessen High School in 1950 and the two joined the Navy in 1950 during the Korean War Effort.

Discharged from service in 1954 and John went to the University of Pittsburgh in Pennsylvania

Married Peggy Ann Poole in 1956 between semesters.

Graduated in 1958 just after the birth of their first son; Jay Durbin Husher

Went to work for Westinghouse Transistor Plant in Youngwood, Pa.

Invented the first silicon integrated amplifier on a single chip in 1959 while personally working during lunch hour. John stopped eating lunch in 1954 since he couldn't afford to eat lunch while in college and hasn't eaten lunch since. Invented the first epitaxial silicon integrated circuit process in 1959.

Wright Patterson Air Base awarded Westinghouse a major contract based on his integrated amplifier and Westinghouse was given an eleven million dollar contract to develop special integrated amplifiers for use in space shots. Westinghouse started a new division based on this called *Molecular Electronics Division (MED)* and built a plant in Baltimore Maryland for the development and production of Integrated Circuits (new name)

A daughter, Karen lynn was born to Peg and John in June of 1960.

A son ,David Todd, was born to Peg and John in April 1962.

John was promoted to Manager of the Custom Products Division. They supplied special integrated circuits for customers such as Univac and the MIT division responsible for the Apollo Space Ship.

John left Westinghouse late in 1965 to join Sprague Electric in Worcester Mass. as the General Manager and Plant Manager for a building being built there to produce integrated circuits which Sprague didn't produce at the time. They successfully built the first complete laminar flow production area in 1966-67 and produced their first integrated circuits in 1967.

John left Sprague late in 1968 to join Fairchild Semiconductor in Mountain View Ca. to become the Director of Digital Integrated Circuits – responsible for engineering and production in South Portland Maine, Shiprock New Mexico, Mountain View Ca., and to establish a plant in Singapore for the production of digital integrated circuits

John became the Director of Fairchild Linear Integrated Circuits in 1971.

John left Fairchild in 1982 to become the Vice President and General Manager for Micrel Semiconductor in 1982.

John retired from Micrel after twenty years as VP and GM in 2002 at the age of 70.

John wrote and had published ten books from 2006 through 2009. Six were nonfiction and four were fiction – none about his work.

John's wife Peg passed away June 28 2010 after 54 years of marriage.

John wrote no more books until this present book *Life and Death* in 2015 at the age of 83. He is writing the fourth book of the nonfiction series at this time.

# References and Credits

1. http://www.livescience.com/23989-human-life-span-jump-century.html
2. http://www.halinaking.co.uk/Location/Yorkshire/Frames/History/1315 Great Famine
3. http://en.wikipedia.org/wiki/Great Famine of 1315-17
4. En.wikipedia.org/wiki/Photosynthesis;R.E.Blankenship.okfirst.ocs.ou.edu/train/meteorology/EnergyBudget2.html
5. http://www.vlib.us/mediieval/lectures/black-death.html
6. http://en.wikipedia.org/wiki/Black-Death
7. http://en.wikipedia.org/wiki/earth
8. http://en.wikipedia.org/wiki/Earth
9. http://www.archives.gov/exhibits/influenza-epidemic
10. http://www.archives.gov/exhibits/influenza-epidemic
11. http://www.archives.gov/exhibits/influenza-epidemic
12. http://en.wikipedia.org/wiki/United-States-Pacific Fleet
13. http://en.wikipedia.org/wiki/World-War-II
14. http://en.wikipedia.org/wiki/World-War-II
15. End of smallpox. http://en.wikipedia.org/wiki/Smallpox
16. https://www.johnmuirhealth.com/custom/sem-gynecologic-cancer-service
17. http://downloaded.aol.com/article/2015/03/26/what we can all learn from Angelina jollies-op-ed/21158146/?icid=maing-rid7%7Chtmlws-m
18. www.HealthLetter-MayoClinic.com
19. http://downloaded.aol.com/article/2015/03/26/what-we-can-all-learn-from-angelina-jolies-op-ed/21158146/?icid=maing-grid7i%7Chtmlws-m.
20. April 2015 Bottom Line/Health
21. http://en.wikipedia.org/wiki/Black_Death
22. http://en.wikipedia.org/wiki/Cholera

23. http://en.wikipedia.org/wiki/Anthrax
24. http://dermatology.about.com/cs/smallpox/a/smallpoxhx.htm
25. http://en.wikipedia.org/wiki/Spanish_flu
26. http://en.wikipedia.org/wiki/Printing_press
27. Microbe Hunters by Paul De Kruif, Introduction copyright 1996 by Harcourt, Inc. A Harvest Book Harcourt, Inc.
28. http://www.ucmp.berkeley.edu/history/hooke.html
29. http://inventors.about.com/od/mstartinventions/a/microscope.htm
30. http://en.wikipedia.org/wiki/Ilya_Ilyich_Mechnikov
31. http://en.wikipedia.org/wiki/Oxygen
32. http://en.wikipedia.org/wiki/Theobald_Smith
33. http://www.1911encyclopedia.org/Sir_David_Bruce
34. http://nobelprize.org/nobel_prizes/medicine/laureates/1902/ross-bio.html
35. http://www.mcatmaster.com/medicine&war/yellowfever.htm
36. http://www.britannica.com/eb/article-9032103/Paul-Ehrlich
37. http://en.wikipedia.org/wiki/Joseph_Lister
38. http://www.emc.maricopa.edu/faculty/farabee/BIOBK/BioBookgenintro.html
39. http://en.wikipedia.org/wiki/Charles_Darwin
40. http://www.haciendapub.com/faria5html
41. The Demon Under the Microscope, by Thomas Hager, published by Harmony Books, an imprint of the Crown Publishing Group, a division of Random House, Inc., New York in 2006
42. http://en.wikipedia.org/wiki/Sulfonamide_(medicine)
43. http://inventors.about.com/od/pstartinventions/a/Penicillin.htm
44. The Mold in Dr. Florey's Coat by Eric Lax, published by Henry Holt and Company 2004
45. http://en.cellsalive.com/pen.htm
46. http://en.wikipedia.org/wiki/Gram-negative
47. Splendid Solution: Jonas Salk and the Conquest of Polio/Jeffrey Kluger, published by The Berkley Publishing Group, The Penguin Group
48. http://homepage.smc.edu/hgp/history.htm
49. http://en.wikipedia.org/wiki/Amino_acid
50. The Genetic Code by Isaac Asimov, published by The New American Library, Inc., 1962
51. http://en.wikipedia.org/wiki/DNA

52. The Double Helix by James D. Watson, published by TOUCHSTONE, First Touchstone Edition, 2001
53. How Did We Find Out About DNA? By Isaac Asimov, published by Walker and Company, New York, 1985
54. http://www.estrellamountain.edu/faculty/farabhee/biobk/ BioBookPROTS Yn.html
55. http://en.wikipedia.org/wiki/Chromosome
56. http://en.wikipedia.org/wiki/Human_Genome_Project
57. http://en.wikipedia.org/wiki/Genetic_code
58. http://en.wikipedia.org/wiki/Retrovirus
59. **http://en.wikipedia.org/wiki/AIDS**
60. http://stemcell.nih.gov/info/basics/basics1.asp
61. http://en.wikipedia.org/wiki/HIV
62. http://en.wikipedia.org/wiki/Base_pair
63. http://en.wikipedia.org/wiki/Cell_(biology)
64. Internet article titled Temperature by John Baez.
65. Robert Koch Biography; *Nobel Lectures, Physiology or Medicine 1901-1921*, Elsevier Publishing Company, Amsterdam, 1967
66. www.bio-**medicine**.org/tag/**SARS**/ - 29k
67. *Nature Medicine* published an article in September 2006, authored by Menno de Jong
68. en.wikipedia.org/wiki/**Ebola** - 125k
69. en.wikipedia.org/wiki/**HIV** - 261k
70. en.wikipedia.org/wiki/History_of_the_**alphabet** - 115k
71. en.wikipedia.org/wiki/Gregor_**Mendel** - 51k
72. users.adelphia.net/~lubehawk/BioHELP!/**mendel**.htm - 96k
73. en.wikipedia.org/wiki/**Mendelian**_inheritance - 44k
74. en.wikipedia.org/wiki/**Inception**_of_**Darwin**'s_**theory** - 91k
75. en.wikipedia.org/wiki/The_**Origin**_of_**Species** - 157k
76. en.wikipedia.org/wiki/**Oliver_Wendell_Holmes** Sr. - 42k
77. content.nejm.org/cgi/content/full/343/8/587
78. en.wikipedia.org/wiki/Gerhard_**Domagk** - 35k
79. www.chemsoc.org/timeline/pages/1928.html - 36k
80. en.wikipedia.org/wiki/**Legionella** - 53k
81. en.wikipedia.org/wiki/Acetic_**acid_bacteria** - 23k
82. medic.med.uth.tmc.edu/path/00001497.htm - 3k
83. en.wikipedia.org/wiki/**Penicillin** - 79k
84. www.geocities.com/Athens/Ithaca/2155/**history**.htm - 6k

85. www.eyewitnesstohistory.com/plague.htm - 29k

86. www3.baylor.edu/~Charles_Kemp/**typhus**.htm - 7k

87. www.ideafinder.com/history/invention**s**/print**press**.htm - 61k

88. **Hunt**-for-**Chromosomal**-Errors-Which-Cause-Genetic-Diseases-11203-1/ -

89. deHaseth P. Helmann (1995). "Open complex formation by Escherichia coli RNA polymerase: the mechanism of polymerase-induced strand separation of double helical DNA".

90. from Purves et al., *Life: The Science of Biology*, 4ᵗʰ Edition, by Sinauer Associates (www.sinauer.com) and W. H. Freeman (www.whfreeman.com). Used with permission.

91. Image from Purves et al., *Life: The Science of Biology*, 4ᵗʰ Edition, by Sinauer Associates.
(www.sinauer.com) and W. H. Freeman (www.whfreeman.com). Used with permission.

92. http://en.wikipedia.org/wiki/Bone_marrow_transplant

93. BottomLineHealth.com, April 2015

94. **Stem Cell of America** about the use of stem cells for multiple sclerosis

95. *Harvard Heart Letter*, April 2015

96. *Health & Nutrition Letter*, 2015

97. BottomLineHealth.com, April 2015

98. www.health.harvard.edu, April 2015

99. Healthafter50, April 2015

100. *Time*, April 6, 2015

101. *Bottom Line Health,* April 2015

102. www.health.harvard.edu *Harvard Health Letter*, April 2015

103. http://www.closerlookatstemcells.org/Top=Stem-Cell-Treatment-Facts.html

104. http://bit.ly/bn9der

105. *Bottom Line Personal*, April 2015